Test-Driving Complementary Therapies

Sylvia Thompson

Dr Muiris Houston

Newleaf

Newleaf
an imprint of
Gill & Macmillan Ltd
Hume Avenue, Park West
Dublin 12
with associated companies throughout the world
www.gillmacmillan.ie

© Sylvia Thompson 2002
0 7171 3282 X
Design by Vermillion
Print origination by Linda Kelly
Printed by ColourBooks Ltd, Dublin

This book is typeset in Stone Informal 9pt on 14pt.

The paper used in this book comes from the wood pulp of managed forests. For every tree felled, at least one tree is planted, thereby renewing natural resources.

A CIP catalogue record for this book is available from the British Library.

1 3 5 4 2

Contents

CONTENTS

Acknowledgments

Writing this book has been a great pleasure. I would first like to thank Sheila Wayman, Features Editor at *The Irish Times* for commissioning me to write the series, Alternative Agenda, without which this book wouldn't exist. Secondly, I would like to thank Eveleen Coyle, my editor at Gill & Macmillan, who showed great enthusiasm for the project right from the start. In writing the medical views of each therapy, Dr Muiris Houston, Medical Correspondent with *The Irish Times* placed alternative therapies in the context of orthodox medicine. For his contribution, I am very grateful.

Test-Driving Complementary Therapies would also never have made it to the printers if those who tested out the therapies and those who advocated them in the original *Irish Times* series were not willing to have their accounts published in book form. I would like to thank friends, colleagues and family members who acted as guinea pigs by accepting my request to try out a therapy and report back on the experience. Also, I am indebted to those who came forward to tell me how a certain therapy helped them through a time of emotional difficulty or physical illness. These accounts provide a valuable insight into recovering good health and well-being which cannot always be quantified and statistically analysed.

On a personal note, I would like to sincerely thank my family and in particular: my sister-in-law, Kay Neill, who lovingly looked after my children while I strove to meet a fast-approaching deadline; my daughters, Kaitlin and Beulah, for their love and inspiration; my parents, Cecil and Nellie, whose open-mindedness on health matters was a formative influence, and finally my husband, Des Fox, who patiently listened (at least, I think he was listening) while I was working on this book. For someone who is himself brimful with ideas, I am truly grateful to him for his valuable feedback throughout the writing of *Test-Driving Complementary Therapies.*

Introduction

A clogged-up healthcare system. Over busy GPs. Long waiting lists for specialist medical care. Crowded outpatient departments and hospitals. Overtired interns and nurses pushed to their limits.

This is the backdrop that has led many individuals to search out alternative approaches to solve their health problems. Some people find a therapy that suits them. They respond well to treatment and regain good health, with a new sense of power and responsibility to look after themselves.

However, other people set out in their search for alternatives, uneducated about their choices and the pitfalls that might await them (e.g. under-qualified or unregistered practitioners, incorrect diagnoses, inappropriate treatment). These individuals, although looking for a more personal approach to their problem and a longer-term solution, can founder in a sea of unknowns. They don't really know what acupuncture is all about. They don't understand the principles of homeopathy or herbalism. They are confused by contradictory nutritional advice. They are fearful of chiropractic or osteopathic manipulation, yet sense it might help them. This book is for these people.

It is the compilation of a series of articles that appeared weekly in *The Irish Times* in 2000. The series was called the Alternative Agenda and the response to it from the public was huge. Many readers followed the series week by week, taking clippings of their favourite therapies. Others contacted *The Irish Times* for back issues of the paper on days they didn't get it.

Many readers spoke to me personally about how they particularly enjoyed the question and answer format of the articles. Each therapy was approached with the same format: What is it? What does it treat? A first-timer's experience; An advocate's view and The medical view. As the series drew to a close, the idea for a book was born.

In *Test-Driving Complementary Therapies*, I have kept to the same format as the articles, and people who tried out therapies and advocated them have kindly given me their permission to use their accounts in the book. I have also added information about the origins of each therapy.

Researching the origins of each therapy was fascinating. It gave me an insight into the ancient philosophical and medical systems which are the foundations of many 'alternative' therapies. Reading about systems including the Indian Ayurvedic tradition, traditional Chinese medicine and Ancient Greek, Egyptian, and Roman practices shows how relatively new what we call conventional medicine still is. Some alternative therapies such as Western herbal medicine and homeopathy were in fact the standard practice in some countries before they were replaced by the modern conventional medical approach (also known as allopathic medicine).

Where available, I have also given more comprehensive contact details and websites for the therapies so that *Test-Driving Complementary Therapies* can be a resourceful starting point for people who want to find out more. Choosing a practitioner who is a member of an established register of therapists is of utmost importance. By doing so, you – the client – have a guarantee that the therapist you attend is professionally trained, accredited to a professional body and insured to work in his/her chosen domain. Never make an appointment with a therapist without first checking out his/her credentials. Although there are moves towards statutory regulation for complementary therapies, most professional bodies – like the medical profession itself – are self-regulated.

Nowhere in this book is conventional medicine wilfully undermined. It would be foolish to claim that alternative therapies can now replace a system of medicine which can carry out complex and intricate surgery, offer aggressive treatments to kill cancers and fight infectious disease effectively with strong drugs and vaccines. The medical views of each therapy provided by *Irish Times* medical correspondent Muiris Houston are invaluable because they place the alternatives in the context of the standard conventional medical approach that most of us grew up with.

I believe conventional medicine and alternative or complementary therapies have distinct roles to play in healthcare. Sometimes, alternative therapies can work hand in hand with conventional medical treatment. In other cases, if people respond to their health problems with the help of an alternative practitioner, they can save themselves considerable pain and even surgery. In yet other cases, acute medical intervention is the only option.

As complementary therapies continue to become more and more established, the general public will begin to understand better for which conditions homeopathy, herbalism, acupuncture, chiropractic or osteopathy can be used on their own, as a complement to orthodox medicine or as a tried and trusted alternative. When this time comes, I believe we will have matured in our approach towards genuine good health. Only then can preventative medicine – as advocated by many therapies in this book – truly play a valuable role in our lives.

Acupuncture

What is it?

Acupuncture is a branch of Chinese medicine which uses very fine needles placed at specific points on nerve or energy pathways called meridians. The principle is that chi (energy) moves along these meridians and when blockages occur, pain or illness results. The needles stimulate points along the meridians to reduce or increase the energy flow, remove blockages and tone and restore balance to the system. The addition of heat (called moxibustion) at the acupuncture points is believed to enhance the flow of energy.

What are its origins?

Acupuncture is a branch of traditional Chinese medicine, which dates back over four thousand years. Traditional Chinese medicine is believed to have spread to Japan in the sixth century. Europeans first came into contact with it through French Jesuit missionaries based in Japan.

The Western world was introduced to acupuncture on a wide scale in the early 1970s; a journalist covering the visit of US president Richard Nixon to China had emergency surgery to remove his appendix. The operation was done using acupuncture for pain relief rather than an anaesthetic. The journalist's experience of acupuncture was given worldwide coverage, which led to investigations into its widespread use in Chinese hospitals.

What does it treat?

In theory, virtually any complaint can be treated with acupuncture, although caution should be taken by those suffering from cancer. In practice, it is considered good for relieving pain in the back, shoulder, neck and arms. It is also considered appropriate treatment for asthma, eczema, headaches, menstrual and gastro-intestinal problems. Acupuncture is also sometimes used as a replacement for chemical anaesthetic during surgery, childbirth and dental treatment.

A first-timer's experience

A 35-year-old female journalist

With detailed personal and family medical history taken, lifestyle discussed, tongue examined and pulse taken: my treatment began. Squeamish about injections and even the occasional misplaced sewing needle, I was nervous and not at all looking forward to the sensation of the acupuncture needles crossing the subcutaneous layer of my skin. So, I decided not to watch, but I did feel all nine needles as the acupuncturist pierced my skin and twisted the fine needles anti-clockwise (the direction believed to reduce pain) into place along four different energy pathways of my body.

Yes, it does hurt and you do feel the blood rush to the spot when the needle is in place. But, it is a dull pain. While the needles were in position for twenty minutes or so, the acupuncturist burned a *moxa* stick (rolled Chinese herb) around the area most prone to pain. This was a comforting feeling.

Then, once the needles were removed, she oiled the skin of the surrounding areas. A short neck and shoulders massage concluded the one-hour session. I left feeling tingly and exhilarated.

An advocate's view of acupuncture for tennis elbow and back pain

A 50-year-old female public-relations consultant had her first acupuncture treatment six years ago and continues to have acupuncture three or four times a year.

I had got to the stage that I couldn't lift a tea cup, my arm was so weak. I had previously had a cortisone injection which worked immediately, but the pain came back again six months later. I went for four or five acupuncture treatments on the advice of my GP. The pain just disappeared.

I work quite a lot at a computer and I don't have very good posture which gives me backache. I now go for acupuncture to relieve this. I use it in a preventative way in that if I get a twinge I don't let it develop. However, I did go for some treatment recently when my back was knotted and my muscles were in spasm and it took away the pain. Basically, I find acupuncture is very relaxing. It doesn't hurt. There are no side effects and it takes away pain and soreness.

The medical view

There is good evidence from randomised trials that there is a greater pain relief from the positioning of needles on recognised acupuncture points than the placing of them just anywhere on the body. However, any research that has been done is hospital-based for acute conditions such as post-operative pain rather than for chronic conditions. That said, there is other evidence that supports the use of acupuncture in pain conditions such as migraine, the treatment of nausea and substance misuse (e.g. drug abuse). Trials of acupuncture in asthma and hay fever produce conflicting results, and acupuncture has not been shown to work for those with tinnitus, obesity or those quitting smoking.

In a study reported in the *British Medical Journal*, acupuncture was found to be an effective short-term treatment for patients with chronic neck pain but there was only limited evidence for long-term effect after five treatments.

Choosing a practitioner

The Irish Acupuncture and Chinese Medicine Organisation can be contacted at tel: 01 4640444; and Celine O'Connor Casey, Secretary of Acupuncture and Chinese Medicine Organisation, Foxgrove House, Rockbarton, Bruff, Co. Limerick, e-mail: celinecasey@eircom.net. There are currently 130 practising acupuncturists affiliated to this body, which requires members to have a minimum of three years' training.

Medical doctors who have an interest in or practise acupuncture can be contacted via the Irish Medical Acupuncture Society. Tel: 01 2887671.

The British Acupuncture Council has approximately 2,100 members in the UK. You can obtain contact details of their register from 63 Jeddo Road, London W12 9HQ. Tel: 020 8735 0400. E-mail: info@acupuncture.org.uk.

The British Medical Acupuncture Society is a group of medically qualified doctors who have an interest in or practice acupuncture. It has over 2,000 members in the UK. Members can be contacted through the BMAS at 12 Marbury House, Higher Whitley, Warrington, Cheshire WA4 4QW. Tel: 01925 730727. E-mail: admin@medical-acupuncture.org.uk.

The Acupuncture Association of Chartered Physiotherapists in the UK can be contacted on tel: 01747 861151.

Cost of treatment

A single acupuncture treatment costs between €13/£10 and €130/£100.

BUPA Ireland subsidises treatments by registered acupuncturists. VHI subsidises treatments by GPs who practise acupuncture.

Various health insurance companies in Britain (including ACTPlan, BHSF, HSF and Leeds Hospitals Fund, Legal and General Healthcare, OHRA, Sovereign and Medisure from Sun Alliance) offer contributions towards the cost of acupuncture treatments.

Useful websites
www.acupuncture.org.uk
www.medical-acupuncture.co.uk

Alexander Technique

What is it?

The Alexander Technique is not a therapy as such. Instead it is a process of re-education during which the individual unlearns poor posture and movement that has led to tension and sometimes pain in the body. By becoming consciously aware of the strain and unnecessary effort this is putting on the body, the individual goes on to relearn the body's natural and correct posture and movements.

Alexander Technique teachers focus on teaching people how to release unnecessary tension in their bodies while doing everyday activities such as brushing their teeth, sitting eating at the table, sitting at a desk, standing in a queue, driving a car and walking.

What are its origins?

The Alexander Technique was developed in the late nineteenth century by Australian actor Frederick Matthias Alexander. During performances he began to lose his voice. Alexander observed himself with the use of mirrors and found that he had a habit of pulling his head backwards and downwards before delivering his lines. This movement, he discovered, compressed his spine, chest and ribs. By focussing on lengthening his neck muscles, Alexander regained his voice control.

He went on to explore how rethinking and relearning movements could help numerous other problems. He began to teach his technique, first in London and then in the United States. The Alexander Technique is still widely taught to students of acting, dance and music.

What does it treat?

The Alexander Technique does not treat specific conditions directly; however by unlearning postural errors and becoming consciously aware of the need for good posture, individuals can find relief from back, neck and shoulder pain, tension headaches and repetitive strain injury (RSI). Conditions such as irritable bowel syndrome, asthma, hyperventilation and other breathing difficulties can also be helped with the Alexander Technique.

A first-timer's experience

A 35-year-old female journalist

The calm, slow speaking voice and gentle, controlled body movement of the Alexander Technique teacher (they are not called therapists) was a striking introduction to this consultation. I had come with subtle, achy pains in my arms and a real feeling that if I didn't consciously improve my posture, I would end up with more serious – possibly constant – pain.

The teacher began by asking me about the pain and when it began. He then spoke quite a bit about how we abuse our bodies by bringing tension into certain areas unnecessarily. He demonstrated how we often lock our whole bodies into position when sitting looking at a computer screen rather than keeping our body aligned and simply using our eyes to look at the screen.

He listened carefully as I spoke about my postural mistakes and agreed things like wrist pads in front of keyboards and phone headsets would help. He then observed me while I sat on a chair and stood up from sitting, asking me to place my arm on the back of my head to feel how the muscles in my neck were moving as I did this. He watched me walk around the room, placing his hand on the top of my head to prevent me from tensing it unnecessarily as I walked. Walking like this felt less strained. He also stood behind me and repeated a few words about extending my head upwards and my shoulders downwards to allow my body to extend to its full length and width.

We spoke about how important it is to become aware of one's grip on toothbrushes, knives, forks and pens; how we often create excess tension with unnecessarily tight grips. I left the half-hour session feeling the need to become more conscious about how I do things. I also understood that it would probably take a few more classes (or a lot of conscious effort and checking in the mirror) before I could genuinely unlearn some of my bad habits.

An advocate's view of the Alexander Technique for back pain
A 54-year-old male broadcaster and journalist
I had chronic back trouble for up to twenty years which was related to a football injury. Often my back would go into spasm which would put me in serious pain. I tried everything from acupuncture to chiropractic. I even had surgery which involved the removal of two discs, but this was never completely satisfactory.

Then, I went to an Alexander Technique teacher. He taught me how to walk correctly and how to sit down correctly. He explained to me about the weight of my head on my body and made me aware of the importance of good posture and how to have conscious control of it.

At first, learning these things was hard work. Now it has become habit and I understand that the way I walk and sit are fundamental to how my back feels. I have had a long period of remission from my back problem, but if I get chronic pain again, I will go back to the Alexander Technique teacher. Of all the therapies I tried, none of them have been as good as the Alexander Technique.

The medical view

The Alexander Technique is an accepted method of preventative treatment in back pain. Some doctors and physiotherapists with special training in orthopaedic medicine use the technique as part of an overall treatment plan. It is important to have persistent or recurrent back pain investigated before submitting to any alternative treatments.

Choosing a practitioner

There are 850 teachers of the Alexander Technique in the UK and eight teachers in Ireland. Teachers of the Alexander Technique should have completed a three-year full-time course approved by the Society of Teachers of the Alexander Technique (STAT). Qualified teachers will have the letters MSTAT after their names.

A full list of teachers in the UK and Ireland is available from the Society of Teachers of the Alexander Technique, 129 Camden Mews, London NW1 9AH. Tel: 020 7284 3338.

Cost of treatment

One half-hour/45-minute lesson in the Alexander Technique costs between €26/£20 and €52/£40. A course of between 20 and 30 lessons is usually recommended.

Useful websites

www.stat.org.uk

Aromatherapy

What is it?

Aromatherapy is based on the principle that, when absorbed into the body, a specific mix of highly concentrated distilled plant oils (known as essential oils) can assist in the healing of certain illnesses and ailments. There are approximately 400 essential oils, each with its individual scent or aroma and list of therapeutic properties.

Aromatherapy is one of the most widely used (and some practitioners would say, abused) of all alternative therapies. Adulterated essential oils are often marketed and sold as catch-all cures for all ills.

Aromatherapists use the oils blended together and diluted with a carrier vegetable oil for massage, inhalation and bathing. Massage is considered to be the most effective form of the therapy. In addition to the beneficial effects of the oils, the massage techniques relax the muscular and nervous systems and stimulate the blood and lymphatic systems.

What are its origins?

The medicinal use of plant oils dates back to ancient China. Such knowledge is believed to have reached the West through the Greeks and the Romans. Plant oils were widely used as perfumes, antiseptics and medicines in Britain from the thirteenth to the nineteenth centuries.

The introduction of cheaper chemical copies then replaced essential oils until a revival of interest in natural treatments at the beginning of the twentieth century encouraged their use again. French chemist Professor René Gattefosse is credited with re-introducing them. Later, his work was built on by French physician Dr Jean Valnet and Marguerite Maury, a French biochemist and beautician.

What does it treat?
Aromatherapy is best suited to stress-related disorders, such as digestive problems, fatigue, insomnia, tension headaches, fluid retention, anxiety and mild depression. However, it is also used as a treatment for flu, colds, chronic fatigue, neck and back pain, repetitive strain injury (RSI), menopausal and menstrual complaints.

Some essential oils are not suitable for use during pregnancy. People with diabetes, epilepsy and heart conditions must also avoid certain essential oils. Some essential oils may cause an allergic reaction. Aromatherapy should not be used in conjunction with homeopathic remedies as the essential oils may counteract the homeopathic action.

A first-timer's experience of aromatherapy massage
A 35-year-old female journalist
For this treatment, you need to be relatively comfortable with your body, because, yes, you do have to take off all your clothes except your underpants. After taking my medical history, the therapist left me alone to undress and lie on my back on her couch. The room was warm, softly lit but a little bit stuffy. Upon her return, the aromatherapist made up a blend of oils checking with me on whether I disliked the smell of any one essential before she added it.

Then, oils ready, she began with gentle repetitive strokes down my back. Gradually, she changed the massage stroke and worked into any knobbly areas firmly, yet never causing pain. Then, she moved on to my arms and hands, neck, head, face, legs and finally feet. She covered me completely in towels and left me alone for a few minutes.

Clothes back on and feeling very oily, I returned to the busy city street. I felt relaxed both mentally and physically afterwards. I drank up to three glasses of water throughout the evening (as recommended) and slept well that night.

An advocate's view of aromatherapy for stress relief
A 27-year-old woman working in publishing
My job is quite stressful and at the time, I felt very run-down and tired all the time. I was obsessed with detail and a worrier, although I appeared fine. I went from being an erratic sleeper to a downright insomniac. So, I decided I'd treat myself.

Following a thorough first consultation, I had a series of six treatments. Now, I have a treatment about once a month. I find full-body aromatherapy massage rebalances me. Following the initial six sessions, my sleep problems disappeared.

I find the treatment itself completely relaxing and calming. I forget about everything while I am there. I'm like a zombie afterwards. I just go home and sleep really well that night. Then, for about a week afterwards, I have loads of energy.

The medical view
Aromatherapy oils are said to act both pharmacologically, that is like a drug absorbed into the blood stream through the skin and by olfactory stimulation. Most clinical trials of massage have focussed on the psychological outcomes of treatment. There is good evidence from randomised trials to indicate that massage reduces anxiety scores in the short term in settings as varied as

intensive care, psychiatric institutions, hospices and occupational health. Practitioners and patients report that massage improves self-image in terminal illness.

There are very few clinical trials showing that any massage technique can have specific effects on conditions such as osteoarthritis, epilepsy, infertility or diabetes. There is a need for large-scale randomised trials to assess the use of aromatherapy in chronic health conditions. Although essential oils are pharmacologically active, the lack of a formal reporting scheme for adverse effects in aromatherapy means that the safety of essential oils has not been conclusively established.

Choosing a practitioner
Qualifications held by practising aromatherapists vary hugely from the International Therapy Examinations Council (ITEC) certificates held by beauty therapists who include aromatherapy massage in their portfolio of treatments to the 220-hour minimum training required for members of the Register of Qualified Aromatherapists.

The International Federation of Professional Aromatherapists has over four thousand aromatherapists on its register. They can be contacted via 82 Ashby Road, Hinchley, Leicestershire LE10 1JN. Tel: 01455 637987.

Many aromatherapists in Ireland are members of the Irish and International Aromotherapy Association, 22 St Brigid's Terrace, Mullingar, Co. Westmeath. Tel: 044 42270.

Other aromatherapists in Ireland and the UK are members of one of the 10 professional associations affiliated to the Aromatherapy Organisations Council (AOC), PO Box 19834, London SE25 6WF. Tel: 020 8251 7912.

Many qualified massage therapists and reflexologists also use essential oils. Before booking a treatment, it is advisable to check that the aromatherapist is a member of an association affiliated to the AOC and has professional insurance.

Cost of treatment

Treatments cost between €26/£20 and €65/£50.

Useful websites

www.aocuk.net

Bio-energy Therapy

What is it?

Bio-energy healing is based on the premise that each individual is surrounded by an electromagnetic field of energy known as the aura. Bio-energy therapists work to clear any blockages in this energy as it flows in and out of our bodies through seven energy centres, known as the chakras. It is largely a hands-off therapy, although there may be some laying on of hands.

What are its origins?

In principle, bio-energy therapy dates back to ancient China and the belief that we are all surrounded by a lifeforce energy or chi. Bio-energy therapy as it is practised in Ireland comes from a system of techniques developed by Zdenko Domancic in former Yugoslavia during the 1980s.

What does it treat?

Bio-energy healing is a complementary therapy and not an alternative to medical advice. Clients have noted improvements in asthma, arthritis, backache, insomnia, migraine and tension headaches, depression, anxiety, allergies and skin conditions. It is not recommended for anyone who has a pacemaker because 'energy' changes can cause arrhythmia (irregular heartbeats).

A first-timer's experience
A 40-year-old male artist

The session began with the therapist asking me a little bit about myself – my view of my state of health, my work and my outlook on life. The environment was relaxing. She then explained a little about bio-energy and how it involved checking and restoring the chakras (energy centres of the body). As I had done t'ai chi for a while years ago, I understood something about the chakras.

Then, she asked me to take my shoes off and stand on a mat. She began to do hand movements around my body. She suggested that I think about being in a beautiful place which wasn't difficult as there was birdsong music playing in the background. During this time, she said she was feeling the strength of my energy centres. I felt very relaxed.

About fifteen minutes later, she asked me to sit on a reclining chair. She did more hand movements – both fluttering gestures with her fingers and spiral movements with her palms, sometimes touching points of my body. There was a feeling of time being suspended.

Afterwards, she commented on a shoulder injury which I hadn't mentioned to her. She also made a few other observations. I came out of the one-hour session feeling very calm. I felt the whole thing had quite a charming mystique about it, far removed from therapies such as chiropractic which I have had for back pain. By 10 p.m that same evening, I felt very tired as the therapist had said I might. She recommended that I drink one litre of water in the 24 hours following the treatment.

An advocate's view of bio-energy for back pain
A 46-year-old female executive officer in the civil service

I had suffered from back pain on and off for up to twenty years. I had received treatment from doctors and specialists which helped on the short term, but nothing they did ever sorted it out. I came across bio-energy healing at the annual Mind, Body and Spirit Fair at the RDS, Dublin. I tried it out there and could feel heat and energy in my back.

Later that year, when my back got bad again, I decided to give it a proper try. I had been attending an osteopath for a couple of years up to that but seemed to need more and more sessions to gain any relief. I had difficulty walking by this time and was on prescription painkillers. The bio-energy healer explained to me that all my energy was coming down from my head and was compacting around my lower back area, thus manifesting in the physical pain.

I began to feel better even after the first session and was completely back to normal after about five or six sessions and off all painkillers from then to now. I could do all the things that everyone else takes for granted. Now, three years later, my back is still much better. Looking back now, it appears that for me anyway manipulation alone wouldn't have solved my back problem if the energies around my back weren't aligned.

Now, I sometimes go for a bio-energy session just for general well-being, but if I do get a twinge in my back, I make an appointment straightaway and this keeps it sorted.

The medical view
There is no research evidence for the specific disease benefits of bio-energy therapy. It should certainly never be used as a substitute for the conventional treatment of the conditions it claims to improve. As with all alternative treatments, there may be non-specific benefits for patient well-being which could be attributed to the placebo effect.

Choosing a practitioner
There are approximately 200 therapists practising bio-energy in Ireland and many of them practise other therapies alongside bio-

energy. The Bio-Energy Therapist Association (BETA) in Ireland is the registration body for qualified therapists. Tel: 01 2889919. There is no independent bio-energy therapist organisation in the UK.

Cost of treatment

A one-hour session of bio-energy costs between €39/£30 and €60/£45.

Useful websites

www.complementaryhealth

Bowen Technique

What is it?

The Bowen Technique is a hands-on non-manipulative therapy. It involves the practitioner rolling the muscle and connective tissue on various parts of the patient's body. The thumbs and fingers are used, but the touch is gentle with little pressure applied.

A feature of the technique is a series of breaks during which no work is done and the patient is not touched. This is believed to give the body an opportunity to respond to the information gradually and begin the process of healing itself. One explanation for the effectiveness of the Bowen Technique is that the body's cells communicate with the brain to initiate repair to the damaged tissue or tendons.

What are its origins?

The Bowen Technique was developed by Tom Bowen, a lay practitioner who treated the aches and pains of his co-workers in a cement works and woollen mill in Geelong, Australia. Due to the success of his treatment, Bowen opened his own clinic in the 1960s and went on to treat up to 250 patients a week with a success rate of about 88 per cent after two to three visits.

The Bowen Technique is now being taught to final year students in osteopathy in Australia. The therapy was first brought to the UK in 1993.

What does it treat?

The Bowen Technique is a complementary therapy and not a substitute for medical advice or treatment. However, practitioners prefer that their clients are not undergoing other treatments at the same time as the Bowen Technique. Back and neck pain, frozen shoulder, tennis elbow, repetitive strain injury (RSI) and other musculo-skeletal disorders are believed to respond well to the Bowen Technique. Practitioners also report success with asthma and other respiratory problems, hay fever, kidney problems, insomnia and arthritis.

A first-timer's experience

A 54-year-old male member of the caring profession

My first reaction to the therapist was that she seemed very relaxed, confident and reassuring. I was asked to fill in a brief form regarding my personal and medical details. Then, I spoke about my particular medical problems and the therapist spoke a little about the Bowen Technique. Following this, I was asked to take off my jacket and shoes and lie on my abdomen on the plinth.

The therapist began to do rolling movements of the muscles on various parts of my body – my ankles, my lower back, my mid back, my shoulders and my neck. After she did some of these rolling actions, she left the room and came back a few minutes later. She explained that these gaps were to allow the healing to begin. During this process, there was beautiful, soothing music playing in the background. The room was warm with a pleasant aroma.

Then, she asked me to lie on my back and repeated the rolling movements with her thumbs and fingers on my ankles, legs, shoulders and neck. After about an hour or so, the treatment was complete.

I felt a bit mystified by the process, wondering how such a simple, gentle movement could effect major change. The therapist emphasised the need to drink plenty of water after the treatment. She advised me that I would need at least three to four sessions to get some real benefit. She also said that I shouldn't participate in any aggressive exercise such as golf or tennis between treatments. I felt relaxed and refreshed afterwards.

An advocate's view of Bowen Technique and frozen shoulder
A 50-something mother of two grown-up children

Six years ago, I developed a pain in my left arm which my GP diagnosed as tendonitis. Following a course of anti-inflammatories, I was given a cortisone injection into my left shoulder. Six months later, the pain started again and I was given another cortisone injection. This time, I got very little pain relief and I decided to go to a chiropractor. Following several treatments, the pain eased but I had to continue exercises so that my shoulder would not freeze up again. After further protracted visits to the chiropractor, the problem eventually healed.

Later, I developed similar symptoms in my right shoulder. I went back to the chiropractor, but this time my shoulder didn't repair following more protracted treatment. Around this time, I read about the Bowen Technique and became very interested in it. I found a Bowen therapist and began to go to her. In fact, two years later, I am still going once a fortnight. It has been absolutely fantastic. She has worked on both my arms and shoulders. Each treatment gives me a great sense of calm.

I believe the treatment taps into your whole body, sending messages to the brain to repair damaged tissue. It has also had a great effect on my bowels and digestive system, which are good barometers of how you are feeling. I also sleep better. Really, I am very happy to have discovered the Bowen Technique. I believe everybody needs a 'little bit of Bowen'.

The medical view

There is considerable evidence from randomised controlled trials of the effectiveness of all types of manipulation for back and neck pain. A specific randomised trial looking at the Bowen Technique for frozen shoulder has demonstrated an improvement of 23 degrees in the range of movement of the shoulder joint in the treatment group. Overall, 67 per cent of patients in the trial showed a significant level of improvement in their symptoms.

Choosing a practitioner

There are 265 qualified practitioners of the Bowen Technique in the UK, including three in Northern Ireland. There are five in Ireland. Therapists in the UK and Ireland can be contacted via the Bowen Therapists European Register. Tel: 076591 20440. Members will have MBTER after their name.

Cost of treatment

One-hour session with a Bowen Technique therapist costs from €26/£20 to €130/£100.

Useful websites

www.thebowentechnique.com
www.bowen-technique.co.uk
www.bowentherapists.com

Buteyko Method

What is it?

The Buteyko Method involves the individual learning a new pattern of shallow breathing through a series of exercises. The principle behind the technique is that asthmatics and sufferers of other breathing conditions such as hyperventilation (over breathing which can result in panic attacks) deplete their stocks of carbon dioxide by over breathing and thus exhaling valuable carbon dioxide.

Carbon dioxide is required to move oxygen from the blood into the cells and tissues of the body and most of the air around us contains a much smaller proportion of carbon dioxide. Shallow breathing increases the amount of carbon dioxide in the body which in turn oxygenates the cells and tissues of the body.

What are its origins?

The Buteyko Method was developed by a Russian professor of physiology, Professor Konstantin Buteyko, fifty years ago. From studies of hundreds of patients, Buteyko developed a theory that much ill health was the result of the body's defence mechanisms trying to compensate for the lack of oxygen.

He observed that patients with cardiac problems, allergies and breathing disorders breathed more than normal and concluded that deep breathing was not just a symptom but a cause of their ailments. A student of Buteyko, Alexander (Sasha) Stalmatski, brought the technique to the West in 1990, working for six years in Australia before moving to London.

What does it treat?

Although primarily used as a treatment for asthma in this part of the world, the Buteyko Method has also been used to treat high blood pressure, heart conditions, eczema, diabetes, migraine, hay fever and other allergies. It has also shown some success in helping people to stop snoring. Practitioners believe that children with asthma, who do not have a lifetime of bad habits to unlearn, may achieve results more quickly. The Buteyko Method is not suitable for anyone suffering from the acute stage of an infectious disease.

A first-timer's experience
A 38-year-old artist and mother of two

The session began with the Buteyko Method teacher asking me for a history of my asthma as well as taking my general medical history. I also filled in a questionnaire on my current state of health – both physical and psychological. I am just recovering from a bad chest infection and my breathing hasn't been great for quite a while. Filling in this questionnaire confirmed for me quite how bad I have been feeling.

The Buteyko Method teacher then explained the method to me. He explained how when they feel out of breath, asthmatics often begin to hyperventilate in an effort to gulp air. Instead, the idea behind Buteyko is to stop breathing for an instant, close your mouth and begin breathing through your nose.

Under his instruction, I began to breathe through my nose. I sat on a chair with my hands on my chest, breathing through my nose. My initial reaction was one of panic, but gradually I moved beyond this. Once, I became assured that I could breathe this way,

I found it easier. The Buteyko practitioner said that I was taking about 30 breaths a minute, whereas I really could get by with only two. I felt he understood the asthmatic psyche.

He then went on to show me to how take a pause from breathing by holding my nose. Then, I lay on my back with my knees bent and my hands on my chest. Again, I was shown how to breathe through my nose. By the end of the session, I was a lot more relaxed. I felt I was breathing more easily and that I might return for another session to learn the method more fully.

An advocate's view of the Buteyko Method and asthma
An 11-year-old boy

I first got asthma last October and began taking inhalers (both preventers and relievers). Over the next few months, my doctor said that I was getting better and better, breathing stronger and getting a higher score on the peak-flow monitor. So, I stopped taking my preventer inhaler and only took the reliever when I really had to.

One night when I was in bed, I got a very bad asthma attack and the next day, I got three more attacks. I was very worried and didn't know what to do. I lost my confidence after that. I had no energy and couldn't play football or sing in the choir like I used to.

I went back on my inhalers but also started to learn the Buteyko Method. I learned the different types of breathing and practise them now for about three minutes a day after school. Also, I lie on the floor for 15 minutes with my eyes closed when I come home from school each day. Now, I can keep up with my friends, do my football training and go to my singing rehearsals.

I still take my inhaler (preventer), but I try to do the breathing exercises if I feel an attack coming on. I still take my inhaler (reliever) to football and I may need a puff now and again. But, I feel more confident that I will be able to cut down on my inhaler and do the breathing exercises instead.

The medical view
Asthmatics should never substitute breathing methods for medication. A person with severe asthma who stops taking regular medication could be putting his or her life in danger. The scientific principles behind the Buteyko Method are soundly based. However, I am not aware of published studies proving its efficacy in any medical condition.

Choosing a practitioner
The Buteyko Association of Ireland can be contacted at Ballinvella, Lismore, Co. Waterford, or through Fergal Tobin on tel: 01 4650030. Currently, there are two qualified teachers of the Buteyko Method in Ireland.

There is no national register of Buteyko practitioners in the UK; contact details of Buteyko practitioners are available from Dr Lapa, a practitioner on 020 8944 6959.

Cost of treatment
Sessions cost €65/£50 each and a series of three is recommended initially. Clients can sometimes choose between one-to-one therapy or workshops on the technique. Some therapists offer a money-back guarantee that the patients they treat will experience improvement in their condition.

Useful websites
www.buteyko.co.uk
www.buteyko.com
www.buteyko.org.uk

Traditional Chinese Medicine

What is it?

Traditional Chinese medicine (TCM) is a system of medicine which uses acupuncture, herbs, massage, breathing exercises and nutritional advice to correct imbalances in the patient's physical and emotional health. The various parts of the body are believed to be dependent on one another in order to function healthily. Human beings are also believed to be affected by the rhythms of nature, climatic changes and other environmental factors.

The concept of balance (tao, as it is often called) is at the heart of traditional Chinese medicine with two opposing but complementary forces yin and yang, being central to all diagnosis. Yin qualities are associated with cold, dampness, earth, tranquillity and darkness, while Yang qualities are related to heat, fire, light, restlessness and dryness.

The five elements – fire, earth, metal, wood and water – are also used to describe the body, each element controlling particular organs and body functions. The twelve organs referred to in traditional Chinese medicine diagnosis are not the same as those in Western medicine, yet each has a set of functions, areas of the body it controls and a meridian along which acupuncture points are located. In traditional Chinese medicine, chi means energy or life force. The strength of chi determines our vitality and is the catalyst for all the body processes.

What are its origins?

The practise of traditional Chinese medicine dates back over 4,000 years. Medical texts were created to back up practice 2,500 years ago. Knowledge of traditional Chinese medicine began to reach the West in the fifteenth and sixteenth centuries and some Chinese herbs were first imported to Europe in the sixteenth century.

What does it treat?

Traditional Chinese medicine treats all physical illnesses and infections as well as psychological problems such as depression. A traditional Chinese medicine practitioner will usually combine the use of herbs for specific conditions with acupuncture and nutritional advice.

Chinese herbal medicines are considered to be useful for conditions such as acne, anxiety, asthma and bronchitis, coughs and colds, cystitis, digestive disorders, high blood pressure and poor circulation, insomnia, menstrual and menopausal problems, psoriasis and post-viral syndrome.

A first-timer's experience of traditional Chinese medicine
A 40-year-old film accountant and mother of three

Following some tests I had for a sore knee, I discovered that I had high levels of cholesterol and a poorly functioning liver. I decided I would tackle these problems with traditional Chinese medicine. The visit to the TCM practitioner began with a very thorough interview about my health and lifestyle. She asked me all about my lifestyle, what I ate every day and when.

She told me that in TCM, the liver function is very closely associated with the digestive system. (In traditional Chinese medicine, the liver is referred to as 'gan' and is not the same as the liver referred to in conventional Western medicine). She asked me about my medical history. She checked my eyes, asked whether I could hear my heart beat in my head, examined my tongue and took my pulse. This all took about an hour. Then, she gave me an acupuncture treatment.

She suggested that I try to eat at regular times, chew my food well and not to eat on the hoof – while standing up, watching television or reading. She said that we don't get as much benefit from our food if we are doing other things while we eat. She advised me not to drink anything one hour before eating and to always eat cooked foods in the wintertime (i.e. to eat foods in season).

She suggested I avoid foods with excess sugar, greasy foods, nuts, alcohol, chocolates, bananas and cheese and not to eat more than one pint of dairy foods a day. She said I should eat tofu daily as it contains an easily digestible form of calcium. She also suggested that I get a 20-minute nap in the middle of the day. She said that on my next visit, she would give me some Chinese herbs.

An advocate's view of traditional Chinese medicine for bowel problems

A 35-year-old male office-based professional

I had been taking steroids as part of my treatment for ulcerative colitis or Crohn's Disease (my consultant couldn't decide which I had) when I decided to try Chinese medicine. I was suffering from blood and mucus in my stools and various drug combinations had been tried to no effect. I felt I was putting on weight with the steroids and had less energy. I needed to try something else as well as changing to an immuno-suppressant drug (which was prescribed when I stopped taking the steroids).

When I went to the Chinese medicine practitioner, she advised me on changes in my diet, such as cutting out yeast products, cutting back on dairy foods, eating my main meal in the middle of the day and taking a prescribed food supplement. She defined my problem as a spleen and kidney yang deficiency. She made me up a herbal treatment with 12 different herbs and told me to boil the herbs and drink the infusion three times a day after my meals.

I started to feel better within three days of taking the herbs. Within three weeks, my symptoms had cleared up completely. I've been taking the herbs for six weeks now as well as making changes to my diet and lifestyle and having regular acupuncture. I feel all of these have brought about a significant difference in a short time.

The medical view

There are no randomised controlled trials demonstrating the efficacy of Chinese herbal medicine. Recently, one such treatment was implicated in the development of liver toxicity in a number of patients in the UK. The risks of herbal medicine lie in the possibility of contamination and in the variable nature of dosages. There is also the risk of a drug interaction with conventional medicines.

Choosing a practitioner

The Irish Register of Chinese Herbal Medicine is the main register of Chinese Herbalists in Ireland and is affiliated to the European Herbal Practitioners Association. Members can be contacted through the Secretary, 24 Hamilton St, Dublin 8. Tel: 01 8533043. Many Chinese medicine practitioners are also members of the Irish Acupuncture and Chinese Medicine Organisation. A register of members is available. Tel: 01 4640444. Also Celine O'Connor Casey, Secretary of Acupuncture and Chinese Medicine Organisation, Foxgrove House, Rockbarton, Bruff, Co. Limerick, e-mail: celinecasey@eircom.net.

There are approximately 450 members of the Chinese Herbal Medicine register in the UK. They can be contacted via Office 5, Ferndale Business Centre, 1 Exeter St, Norwich, NR2 4QB. Tel: 01603 623994. E-mail: herbmed@rchm.co.uk.

Cost of treatment

A treatment costs from €26/£20 to €39/£30 and herbal remedies cost from €6.50/£5 per prescription, depending on the herbs required.

Useful websites

www.rchm.co.uk

Chiropractic Manipulation

What is it?

Chiropractic manipulation specialises in treating musculo-skeletal disorders by manipulating the spine and other joints manually. These manipulation techniques are carried out by the chiropractor to improve joint movement, relieve pain, decrease muscle spasm and reduce nerve-root entrapment. The ultimate aim is to return the spinal vertebrae to correct alignment.

Chiropractors may also carry out orthopaedic and neurological tests and observe posture, suggesting ergonomic adjustments and exercises when relevant. X-rays and scans of the spine are sometimes used to assess the damage before treatment begins.

What are its origins?

While spinal manipulation has been around for centuries, modern-day chiropractic was founded by American magnetic healer Daniel David Palmer at the end of the nineteenth century. Palmer believed that if a vertebra is displaced, it may press against nerves and cause an imbalance which results in disease.

One of the basic principles of chiropractic is that pain or dysfunction of an organ or body part can be caused if the spine is not correctly aligned. The word chiropractic is derived from two Greek words, *cheiro* meaning hand and *praktos* meaning to use.

McTimoney chiropractic and McTimoney-Corley chiropractic are gentler versions of chiropractic based on the same principles as standard chiropractic. The technique is named after John McTimoney, a chiropractor who was working in the 1950s. He believed that all parts of the body – the skull, the spine, the pelvis and the limbs – could lose their natural alignment and that gentle actions were sufficient to correct this.

What does it treat?

Chiropractic manipulation is most appropriate for back, neck, shoulder and limb pain. It is also considered suitable for asthma, migraine, psoriasis, diabetes and, perhaps surprisingly, colic in babies. It is not suitable for back pain where there is serious damage to the ligaments, nerve roots or when the spinal cord has been compressed. Nor is it suitable for some forms of arthritis.

A first-timer's experience

A 32-year-old female journalist

My boyfriend had been to a chiropractor so I had some idea that there would be creaking and flexing of joints which might be a little uncomfortable. However, I wasn't prepared for the extent of the creaking and the alarming sound that came when my neck was moved from side to side. It wasn't painful. In fact, it made me laugh and it was all over in an instant.

Before the treatment began, the chiropractor asked me if there was any family history of meningitis, arthritis, rheumatism or if I had had any major operations or accidents. He also asked me about my lifestyle and levels of exercise.

Then, while I was lying fully clothed on the chiropractor's treatment bench, he moved my head from side to side and pushed my shoulder blades down and manipulated some other points on my back where I felt discomfort. He also tested the strength in my arms. Following this, he gave me advice on my posture and position of my desk, phone and computer. He even suggested a place where I should buy a new office seat.

He said I had stiff muscles in my back and that I should place a warm hot-water bottle on my back for 15 minutes or so in the evenings. Immediately after the 20-minute treatment, I felt my neck was a lot freer and a few days later, I feel a lot less discomfort in my back.

An advocate's view of chiropractic and nerve pain
A 32-year-old female sales and marketing executive
I had a viral infection in my lung, which was very painful and made breathing difficult. The doctor prescribed rest and painkillers. After several weeks I still had a constant pain in my left lung and found breathing difficult.

I went to a chiropractor who carried out a scan to assess the condition of my spine which showed areas of extreme tension, hyperactivity, stress and asymmetry in my neck, shoulders and back. The scan also measured nerve flow, showed the degree of pain and monitored the autonomic nervous system, which controls the internal organs.

My chiropractor recommended an intensive care programme starting with sessions three times a week for three weeks, to be followed by a re-evaluation with another scan. I was relieved that there was a logical explanation as to why I felt unwell and that something practical could be done to solve the problem.

Over the following sessions, the chiropractor worked on different parts of my neck, shoulders and back. Each time, he worked on a specific part of my back or neck I felt a clicking sound as the bone moved into place. As part of the corrective process I was given specific exercises to improve my postural and ergonomic movement and a course of joint nutrition supplements.

It takes a while for the body to adapt to its new alignment. I had a car crash a few years ago and was knocked off my bicycle earlier, so much of the damage may date back to these incidents. Directly after the first few treatments, I felt slightly dizzy and sometimes a little emotional. As time went on and my symptoms began to diminish, I felt an energy boost after each treatment. Now, I go about once a month for a checkup to maintain correction. I have also adapted my workstation to improve my posture and decrease the amount of stress on my neck and back.

The medical view
There is substantial evidence from randomised controlled trials of the effectiveness of chiropractic in the treatment of back and neck pain. One trial which took place in a community setting compared routine GP care, physiotherapy and manipulation therapy. Manipulation emerged as superior treatment at the one-year follow up. Further studies are needed to assess the efficacy of chiropractic in the treatment of migraine and asthma, for which treatment benefit has been claimed.

Choosing a practitioner
The Chiropractic Association of Ireland has approximately 70 members, all of whom have qualifications recognised by the International Council of Chiropractic Education. The CAI can be contacted on tel: 044 45525 or at 19 Robinstown, Mullingar, Co. Westmeath. E-mail: mullingarcniro@eircom.net.

The British Chiropractic Association, Blagrave House, 17 Blagrave St, Reading, Berkshire, RG1 1QB has a register of 655 full members. Names and numbers of practitioners in various regions are available on tel: 0118 9505950. E-mail: enquiries@chiropractic-uk.co.uk.

Registered chiropractors will have the letters BSc or MSc or DC after their name.

Cost of treatment

A single treatment costs between €26/£20 and €78/£60. Some chiropractors offer a reduced rate for students and children. Many health insurance companies in the UK and Ireland will offer contributions towards treatments.

Useful websites

www.chiropractic.ie
www.chiropractic-uk.co.uk
www.mctimoney-chiropractic.org

Colonic Hydrotherapy

What is it?

Colonic hydrotherapy is a form of internal detoxification. Purified warm water is flushed gently through the back passage into the colon and the rest of the large intestine and out through a larger tube to clear out accumulated waste matter. Colonic hydrotherapists believe that many illnesses are caused or aggravated by problems in the gut. The premise is that faecal matter containing toxins and bacteria may putrefy and set hard, disrupting bowel function and slowly poisoning the body.

What are its origins?

Colonic hydrotherapy is, in some ways, a more sophisticated and thorough form of an enema. Enemas were once a more commonly used medical procedure, particularly for the treatment of stubborn constipation and before surgical intervention. In 1917, medical doctor John H. Kellogg from Michigan in the USA drew attention to the benefits of colon therapy, as it was first called. His report in the *Journal of the American Medical Association* described how he used it with huge success in the treatment of gastrointestinal disease.

Colon therapy became popular in the 1920s, 1930s and 1940s. From then on up to the 1980s, it was no longer considered a useful treatment. In the last ten years, there has been a resurgence of interest in colonic hydrotherapy among alternative health practitioners.

What does it treat?

Colonic hydrotherapy is a direct treatment for serious constipation, offering immediate relief. Cleaning out the bowel can also help treat irritable bowel syndrome, allergies, candida and yeast infections. Colonic hydrotherapy enables the bowel to be repopulated with so-called friendly bacteria which help control the bacteria which cause intestinal ailments.

Colonic hydrotherapists are very wary of people who want colonic hydrotherapy purely for weight loss. It is also not recommended for those with heart or kidney problems, piles, high blood pressure, bowel cancer or severe diabetes. Neither is it suitable for pregnant women or those who are severely overweight.

A first-timer's experience
A 26-year-old female psychologist

I had read a lot about Western nutrition and the problems it can cause in the colon. These can result in devastating health effects. I believe that there can be huge benefits gained from detoxifying the body. So, it was with this in mind that I went for colon hydrotherapy.

To begin with, I felt I was in safe hands because the therapist was coming from a medical background. She talked to me for about an hour before beginning the treatment and then for about half an hour afterwards. I felt scared of the procedure (which took about 45 minutes) but there is no need for fear. From the point of view of discomfort, the therapist was remarkably good at making sure my dignity was kept intact. There was no pain whatsoever, although I was aware of the procedure. In fact, the sensation of warm and room-temperature water passing through your system is mildly pleasant.

The benefits I gained were not only physical. I would honestly say that I had 300 per cent more energy afterwards. I had a lightness of being and better concentration. But, also I felt released from a lot of stress. Worry and tension seeped away. You clean your teeth, so why not clean your colon?

An advocate's view of colonic hydrotherapy for general well-being
A 43-year-old male complementary health practitioner
I'd been aware of colonic hydrotherapy for a number of years before I tried it. It kept presenting itself as something that would benefit me. Although I didn't have any specific medical complaint, I was not comfortable with my overall level of my health. My energy was low and my digestive system was sluggish.

I began initially with four appointments at weekly intervals. I found colonic hydrotherapy deeply cleansing on a physical level. I felt a great deal lighter physically and mentally after each session and the benefits were cumulative. My digestive system began to function better. Also, it cleared out a lot of emotional detritus – particularly fear – which I believe I held in my gut.

Now, I go for a treatment about once a year. I am aware of the huge mind-body connections and this therapy has been a powerful demonstration of these connections for me.

The medical view
I would be concerned about claims that colon hydrotherapy could prevent colon cancer. Claims that the treatment will help emotional problems and cutting ties that bind are questionable also. Anyone contemplating an invasive therapy such as this should ensure that the practitioner adheres to the highest possible standards of sterilisation and infection control.

Choosing a practitioner
There are about 80 registered practitioners in the UK and Ireland in the Association and Register of Colon Hydrotherapists.

Members can be contacted via 16 Drumond Ride, Tring, Hertfordshire, HP23 5DE. Tel: 0144 2827687. All therapists on the register must have a medical training, a diploma in anatomy and physiology or a recognised qualification in another complementary therapy.

Cost of treatment
A 45-minute session of colonic hydrotherapy costs between €70/£55 and €105/£80.

Useful websites
www.colonic-association.com

Cranio-Sacral Therapy

What is it?

Cranio-sacral therapy is a gentle hands-on therapy that focusses on the flow of the cerebro-spinal fluid throughout the body and in particular from the brain to the base of the spine. This fluid bathes the brain and spinal column and trained cranio-sacral therapists maintain that it creates a rhythmic pulse called the cranial rhythmic impulse.

Disturbances to this rhythm are used in diagnoses and treatment of disorders. Through gentle touch of the cranium and areas along the spinal cord and unwinding movements of the limbs, the flow of the cerebro-spinal fluid is promoted to restore balance, free mobility, release tensions and bring back normal function to an affected area.

What are its origins?

Cranio-sacral therapy grew out of cranial osteopathy which was developed by an American osteopath, Dr William Garner Sutherland (1873-1954). It is based on the premise that the bones in the skull are not fixed but can move slightly. Dr Sutherland showed that – contrary to established medical beliefs – these cranial bones are capable of minute movements and gentle manipulation of them could help adjust the flow of the cerebro-spinal fluid. This in turn would promote healing and rebalancing of the body's systems.

In the 1940s, the first osteopathic school started a post-graduate course in cranial osteopathy. In the mid 1970s, Dr John Upledger was the first practitioner to teach the skills to people who were not trained osteopaths. He coined the phrase cranio-sacral therapy.

What does it treat?
Cranio-sacral therapy is a complementary treatment and not an alternative to medical advice and treatment. Back, neck and shoulder problems, headaches, sinusitis, ear infections, tonsillitis, glue ear, head injuries, temporo-mandibular joint problems, frozen shoulder, arthritis and sciatica are among the conditions most commonly treated with cranio-sacral therapy. It is suitable for all ages, including young children and babies. In children, it is considered useful for treating hyperactivity, dyslexia, learning difficulties and other developmental problems.

A first-timer's experience
A 35-year-old female journalist
The treatment began with the therapist asking me to fill out a form with general personal details and information on any surgery or major accidents I had, any present medication I was taking and if I was attending another health practitioner. He told me that sometimes with cranio-sacral therapy, old injuries may resurface even to the extent of bruising reappearing on the body. Then, he asked me to take off my shoes and socks and lie on my back on the plinth.

He began by gently touching my feet and ankles. He moved to my head, placing his hands on the sides and top of my head and also lifting my head up from my neck and moving it slightly from side to side. He also checked the alignment of my jaws, noting that many people's jaws are out of alignment due to prolonged dental work, which then affects their whole spinal alignment.

Then, he placed one hand under my upper back and touched the area around my chest. He repeated this procedure at my mid back and lower back. He explained how he was tuning into the cerebro-spinal rhythms of my body, checking if there were identifiable areas of imbalance. He said that he could feel that I had a strong level of vitality but that I was somewhat unsettled in myself at the moment (this, I felt was an accurate reading because there is a good deal of change occurring in my life at present).

He then worked on my legs, arms and hands, unwinding my legs at the hips, my arms at the shoulders and my hands at the wrists. Then, he repeated some gentle touching actions and movements on the head and feet before concluding. He left me alone resting for a few minutes on the plinth. We then discussed his assessment of my health.

After the one-hour session, I felt relaxed and happy. Later that evening, I felt I had been energised by the treatment and able to function very well. The therapist said that generally speaking, clients would need up to six sessions at weekly intervals for distinct improvement to a specific condition.

An advocate's view of cranio-sacral therapy for mental and physical exhaustion
A 32-year-old female psychologist

At the end of last year, I was very depleted – both on a physical and an emotional level. I had a plate put in my back following surgery after an accident six years earlier. And, although I appreciated the medical treatment at the time, I was aware that my whole body hadn't been looked after following the accident. I met a cranio-sacral therapist and decided to go for some treatments. I went weekly for about six sessions and now I go on and off.

My energy levels came back up quite quickly following the first few sessions. I also released some emotion that I was holding in my body. I believe that we can hold our emotions in our bodies which was why I had sought out a complementary practitioner, realising that 'talking it out' alone wouldn't suffice. Cranio-sacral therapy is very subtle, gentle and non-invasive and it has worked well for me.

The medical view

There is no evidence to back up claims of the effectiveness of cranio-sacral therapy in learning difficulties, dyslexia, hyperactivity or epilepsy. I would also be cautious about claims that this therapy enables all body tissue to function more effectively.

Choosing a practitioner

There isn't an association of cranio-sacral therapists in Ireland, but there are approximately 15 qualified cranio-sacral therapists working in the country. Tel: 01 8484270 for a list of qualified practitioners.

The International Cranial Association, 478 Baker St, Enfield, Middlesex EN1 3QS, UK, has a list of approximately 100 fully trained cranial osteopaths. Tel: 020 8367 5561.

The Craniosacral Therapy Association at Monomark House, 27 Old Gloucester St, London WC1N 3XX has a register of cranio-sacral therapists. Tel: 01305 268954. E-mail: info@craniosacral.co.uk.

The Craniosacral Society (also the Upledger Institute) at 2 Marshall Place, Perth, Scotland PH2 8AH has a list of cranio-sacral therapists trained at the Upledger Institute. Tel: 01738 444404. E-mail: mail@upledger.co.uk.

Cost of treatment

A one-hour session costs between €32/£25 and €45/£35.

Useful websites
www.craniosacral.co.uk
www.cranio.co.uk
www.craniosacral.org
www.upledger.com

Crystal Therapy

What is it?
Crystal therapy involves the strategic placing of crystals and gemstones on and around the body of the client (who is lying on a plinth) to help rebalance the mental, physical, emotional and spiritual energies in and around them. Each crystal links into one of the seven different chakras or energy centres of the body. The client is also given crystals to hold in his/her hands during the therapeutic session.

What are its origins?
The use of crystals as a source of life and energy is an ancient practice used in healing rituals by shamanic healers in Africa, Australian aborigines and Ancient Egyptians among others. Most ancient philosophies and religions make reference to the magical qualities of crystals, sometimes describing them as gifts from God. Crystal therapy is a revived form of these ancient traditions.

What does it treat?
Different crystals are believed to have different healing properties.

Rose quartz, one of the most popular crystals used in the Western world, is believed to ease fear, guilt, jealousy, anger and resentment. It is also believed to be useful in the treatment of blood disorders and hormonal problems. Other crystals such as amethyst is considered to be a very powerful energiser and blood cleanser and also to enhance intuition and assist meditation. Aquamarine is believed to help banish fears and phobias and is useful for detoxifying the body and reducing fluid.

A first-timer's experience

A 43-year-old female yoga teacher

I went along to the crystal-therapist session with an open mind, although I was somewhat sceptical about the effectiveness of crystals. I've had various healing therapies and although I love the look and feel of crystals, I don't use them.

The crystal therapist took a case history asking me about any physical or emotional health problems. I mentioned three problem areas: breast cysts, lower back pain and sinusitis. She told me about the crystals and what they do. She said that it would be a relaxing therapy and that I would probably fall asleep. As it was my first time, she said that she would give me a balancing and energising treatment.

She asked me to take off my shoes, socks and jewellery and lie on the plinth. She covered me with towels and asked if I needed extra pillows anywhere. She gave me crystals to hold in my hands and made a grid of crystals on and around my body, placing crystals in the region of each of my seven chakras. She talked me through a visualisation process using colour.

I started to become aware that the crystal in my left hand began to feel very heavy and the one in my right hand very light. My stomach was gurgling quite a bit and I became very conscious of the stone on my stomach. It felt warm and very large.

As I went deeper into the experience, I felt my whole body was turning into the shape of a half moon, veering towards the left. I also felt some heat from the stone at my neck. As the session drew to a close, the crystal therapist placed her hands above my forehead and I felt heat from her hands. The visualisation came to an end, she brought me back into the space and gave me time to readjust.

I explained how I had felt and she showed me the stone which she had placed on my stomach. It was about the size of a 10p piece. I was amazed. I couldn't believe it was so small, given how I had felt it so heavy.

She showed me all the stones she had used. And we discussed that my feeling of being dragged to the left might be linked to the fact that I am quite right-brained – disciplined, organised and less emotional. The crystals were drawing me towards my more emotional side. The session lasted about one and a quarter hours in total. The crystal therapist advised me to have a quiet evening following the session and gave me a carnelian stone to keep in my pocket to help with my sinuses.

An advocate's view of crystal therapy for gynaecological problems

A 43-year-old teacher and mother of two

I had suffered with gynaecological problems for two years. Essentially, I had almost continuous menstrual bleeding. During this time I had been given a Depo-Provera injection which failed to alleviate the problem. I subsequently had two D & Cs and a TCRE. The latter has an 85 per cent success rate, but unfortunately it seems that I was one of the other 15 per cent.

About eight months ago, I read about crystal healing on the Internet and I was interested in finding out more. As is the case with many of the alternative treatments (such as acupuncture and reflexology) crystal therapy promotes the natural flow of energy within the body and helps the body's own healing processes. I felt this treatment might be particularly appropriate in my case as the conventional procedures did not seem to be having the desired effect.

I made contact with a crystal healer and set up an appointment. We discussed my problem at length and the healer then began working on me. Since then I have been having crystal therapy once every three to four weeks. Several different types of crystals are used during each session. Rose quartz seems to be particularly appropriate for gynaecological problems, but is very effective for many other complaints also.

After the first couple of sessions, my cycle began to become more regular and has been improving by degrees ever since. I have found crystal healing extremely beneficial as a treatment for my particular problem. I would also recommend it as a very effective form of therapy in terms of general relaxation, well-being and balance.

The medical view
There is no medical or scientific evidence to suggest a health benefit from this form of therapy.

Choosing a practitioner
Jacquie Burgess is probably the best-known crystal therapist practising in Ireland. She can be contacted at Slaney House, Tullow, Co. Carlow. Tel: 0503 51057. E-mail: jacquie@eircom.net. Other crystal therapists in the UK or Ireland can be contacted via the Affiliation of Crystal Healing Organisations, PO Box 100, Exminster, Exeter, Devon EX6 8YE. Tel: 01479 841450.

Cost of treatment
A session can cost between €26/£20 to €52/£40.

Useful websites
www.crystaltherapy.co.uk

Flower Remedies

What is it?

One of the more esoteric alternative therapies, flower remedies are believed to work on an emotional level, helping the body ease itself out of its physical symptoms. The theory behind using them is that flower essences have a vibrational energy of their own which balances the emotions. Emotional imbalance is believed to contribute to many chronic conditions, whereas when the emotions are in balance the body is freer to heal itself.

Bach flower essences, which are one of the most widely used varieties, are obtained by putting the flower heads in spring water and leaving them in the sun. The liquid obtained is preserved in an alcohol solution and bottled.

There are 38 Bach flower remedies, each of which is associated with desired changes in a specific negative emotional state. For example, an essence from the larch flower is given to promote self-esteem and inner confidence, while mimulus flower essence is prescribed for those who have known fears. Other flower essences used today include Californian, Hawaiian and Australian bush flower essence.

Some flower essences are also believed to have an impact on the nervous and immune systems. An anti-viral effect is also associated with some remedies.

What are its origins?

Flower essences have been used for thousands of years in many different cultures. However, the modern-day pioneer of their use is Dr Edward Bach. Practising in the 1930s as a homeopathic doctor, bacteriologist and Harley Street physician, he moved from London to Wales to develop his theories on the healing properties of flowers.

Throughout the 1980s and 1990s, flower essences grew in popularity and are now produced in every continent of the world.

What do they treat?

Flower remedies are not considered to be a substitute for orthodox medical or psychiatric treatment. Instead, they can be used by those who wish to change negative habits, attitudes and ways of behaving, which they believe may be causing stress that may in turn lead to illness. Headaches, insomnia, panic attacks, phobias, anxiety, burn-out, depression are among the problems that flower remedies may help to ease.

Rescue Remedy is by far the best-known mix of flower remedies. It is becoming increasingly popular for its calming qualities following accidents or sudden emotional upheavals.

The remedies come in little dropper bottles and each dose is taken directly on the tongue. Flower remedies are believed to be safe for everyone including babies, children and even animals.

A first-timer's experience

A 39-year-old male designer

I wasn't surprised to learn that flowers might provide remedies for certain conditions and I had taken Rescue Remedy a couple of times. I went along to meet the therapist with an open mind. We began discussing areas of stress in my life.

Surprisingly, I found it incredibly easy to sit and talk with her about my life, even though it was a very informal setting (in a health store). As I spoke about specific areas of difficulty in my work, she seemed to understand quickly which characteristics were blocking my progress.

The philosophy behind the remedies came across as being very respectful of the planet, its beauty and the need for us all to follow our own individual paths through life. After chatting for about an hour, she gave me a list of suggested flower remedies that I could take following another consultation. I went away feeling very pleased to have met someone so inspired by this approach and feel certain that I will try the remedies.

An advocate's view of flower remedies for fearfulness
A 50-year-old senior product consultant with a health food store
I started using Bach flower remedies after my husband died some years ago. I had a lot of things to deal with at that time including being a sole parent. I found the remedies helped me be clearer in myself about what I needed to do. However, it was in connection with my fear of driving that they worked really well for me.

I had always told myself that I couldn't drive but I finally reached the point that I couldn't rely on other people to get me places. I started taking lessons but I was extremely nervous. My driving instructor told me that I was one of the most nervous learners he had ever met. Every time, I put my foot on the clutch, my whole leg trembled and each time I got out of the car, I felt like vomiting.

Then, in consultation with a Bach flower-remedy therapist, I decided I would try to use the flower remedies to help me overcome my fears. I was given a specific mix of remedies linked to feelings of panic, known and unknown fears and the feeling of 'what's the use'. So, I began using them on the spot and took them throughout the day. I decided I would drive home that night and I noticed that my legs weren't trembling.

I continued using the remedies every day, took my driving test and passed on the first attempt. Now, it is two years since I started driving and I still keep a little bottle of flower remedies in my car for use in emergencies. I really believe in them. I think they are wonderful.

The medical view

There is no evidence from randomised controlled trials on the effectiveness of flower remedies. However, usage of such remedies probably has some psychological benefit.

Choosing a practitioner

A list of 1,000 trained Bach flower-remedy therapists in the UK and Ireland is available from the Bach Centre, Mount Vernon, Sotwell, Wallingford, Oxon. OX10 0PZ. Tel: 01491 834678. E-mail: mail@bachcentre.com.

The International Federation of Vibrational Medicine has a list of trained therapists who use a whole range of flower-essence therapies is available from Middle Piccadilly, Holwell, Sherborne, Dorset DT9 5LW. Tel: 01963 250031.

Moira Griffith is one the most experienced therapists working exclusively with Bach flower remedies in Ireland. Tel: 045 865078.

Some other alternative health practitioners advise the use of flower remedies in conjunction with other therapies such as homeopathy, herbalism and aromatherapy. Some psychotherapists also believe they are valuable when used with positive affirmations to promote healthier ways of thinking. Bach flower remedies can be bought in most health-food shops.

Cost of treatment

Treatment costs vary from practitioner to practitioner.

Useful websites

www.bachcentre.com

Homeopathy

What is it?

Homeopathy is based on the principle that like cures like. Minute doses of specially prepared remedies which mimic the symptoms of the illness are given to the patient in the belief that they stimulate deep healing responses.

Homeopaths also prescribe individualised remedies for each patient following a very detailed consultation (lasting up to two hours) on personal and family medical history, diet, emotional well-being and mental alertness. Importance is placed on treating the source of the patient's illness rather than suppressing the symptoms. Symptoms may worsen at first but this is interpreted as heralding improvement.

What are its origins?

The word 'homeopathy' is derived from two Greek words, *homo* meaning like and *pathos* meaning suffering. The law of treating like with like, also called the law of similars, has been part of medical practice since Classical Greek times. Homeopathy as we know it today was first formulated by the German physician and chemist, Samuel Hahnemann, in the early nineteenth century.

What does it treat?

As an alternative to allopathic (conventional) medicine,

homeopathy treats every illness and ailment – physical and/or psychological – as part of an overall imbalance. Chronic illnesses, such as arthritis, asthma, allergies, migraine, digestive and immune disorders, are considered particularly responsive to homeopathy.

Homeopathy is not recommended for surgical emergencies or mechanical dysfunction. It can however be used as a complementary treatment to enhance post-operative healing. Some essential oils used in aromatherapy can interfere with homeopathic remedies.

A first-timer's experience

A 39-year-old teacher and mother of four

I knew a little bit about the format of the consultation so I wasn't surprised that the homeopath spent the whole two hours asking me about every aspect of my life and taking notes. I found the experience very relaxing and therapeutic. I even found myself crying at some points as I recalled certain things.

She asked me about any physical illnesses I had had right back to childhood and if I was taking any medication. She asked me all about my work, my children, any problems they had had and how I was during my pregnancies and during their births. She also left the opportunity wide open for me to comment on other relationships and asked me how I reacted emotionally to difficult situations. She asked me if I had any phobias or recurring dreams.

I was surprised by the level of detail and the level of interest she took in some aspects of my life. She didn't examine me at all. After the consultation, she said she would study her notes and make up a remedy for me. One week later, I got one little tablet sent to me. She said that it wouldn't be an immediate cure and that it was sometimes difficult to get the remedy exactly right the first time. I agreed I would take the tablet at a quiet time and report back to her on how I felt.

An advocate's view of homeopathy for childhood eczema
A mother brought her two-year-old son with severe eczema, sleeplessness and behavioural problems to a homeopath.
Niall was underweight when he was born and had difficulty putting on weight in the first six months of his life. He was a poor feeder and a poor sleeper and a very unhappy child. He had very dry skin from head to toe which developed into eczema. I had used cortisone cream on his skin which improved his eczema, but once I stopped using it, the eczema came back again.

I didn't know anything about homeopathy when my husband and I first brought my son to a homeopath. She asked us absolutely everything about Niall (his feeding, his sleeping, his energy levels, his likes and dislikes, his relationship with his brother and sister), while he sat on the floor beside us playing. She observed him in his play and also asked me about how the pregnancy and birth had been.

She asked us if we would stop using the cortisone cream and use a moisturiser instead. She said that using the cream was not getting to the root of the problem and just suppressing the symptoms. She also said that it was not allowing the body to heal itself and push out the problem which was why Niall's behaviour was so bad. Then, after checking through all her notes, she made up a remedy for Niall.

Within a few weeks, he calmed down a lot. He became less tearful. His skin got worse at first, but because he was less upset, he wasn't scratching it as much. He still didn't sleep well at night. We kept in touch with the homeopath, telling her all this. She then altered his remedy slightly and eventually, he began sleeping through the night. We went to her four times when Niall was two and then before he started playschool and when he started in primary school.

He is now a bright, happy and sociable boy at school. He gets on much better with his sister and brother and his concentration has improved. I feel that he had to be treated as a whole in order for his skin to improve and that his emotional state and behaviour were the root of his problem.

The medical view

Homeopaths prescribe oral medicine, but use a different principle to conventional doctors. Practitioners select a drug that would, if given to a healthy volunteer, cause the presenting symptoms of the patient. This makes it difficult to apply the usual research criteria to prove the efficacy of treatment.

Most research has concentrated on establishing whether homeopathy is a placebo treatment. A recent large-scale analysis in the *Lancet* medical journal concluded that 'the clinical effects of homeopathy are not completely due to the placebo effect'.

There is currently insufficient evidence that homeopathy is effective for any single condition. This includes its use in eczema, for which randomised trials have not been performed.

Choosing a practitioner

Members of the Irish Society of Homeopaths can be contacted at Ruxton Court, 35-37 Dominick St, Galway City. Tel: 091 565040. E-mail: ishom@eircom.net.

The Irish Medical Homeopathic Association is a group of medically trained doctors who take an interest in or practise homeopathy. Tel: 01 2697768.

Members of the Society of Homeopaths in the UK can be contacted at 4a Artizan Road, Northampton NN1 4HU. Tel: 01604 621400. E-mail: info@homeopathy-soh.org.

A list of the 550 members of the Homeopathic Medical Association is available from 6 Livingstone Road, Gravesend, Kent DA12 5DZ. Tel: 01474 560336. E-mail: info@the-hma.org.

Medical doctors, dentists and vets who practise homeopathy can be contacted via the British Homeopathic Association, 15 Clerkenwell Close, London EC1R OAA. Tel: 020 7566 7800. E-mail: info@trusthomoeopathy.org. The BHA has a national directory that includes doctors, dentists, vets and pharmacists who practice homeopathy or dispense homeopathic remedies.

Homeopaths in the UK will have RSHom or FSHom after their name. Homeopaths in Ireland will have ISHom after their name. Medical doctors who have taken post-graduate training in homeopathy use MFHom, FFHom or LFHom.

Cost of treatment
A homeopathic treatment costs between €39/£30 and €105/£80.

Useful websites
www.the-hma.org
www.homeopathy.org

Hypnotherapy

What is it?

Hypnosis is a technique used mainly in psychotherapy to gain access to the roots of many physical and psychological problems. By cutting through the conscious mind – and therefore many of the habits, strategies and inhibitions – with relaxation techniques, the hypnotherapist plants positive suggestions in the subconscious mind of the client to alter negative behaviour patterns, attitudes and habits.

What are its origins?

The use of hypnotic states to heal dates back to ancient times. The Druids called hypnosis 'magic sleep'. The Ancient Greeks and Egyptians had sleep temples for healing. Patients were given curative suggestions while they were in a trance or slept.

Modern hypnosis began with the eighteenth-century Austrian physician, Franz Anton Mesmer, who demonstrated cures using 'animal magnetism'. His technique later became known as Mesmerism. However, hypnosis did not gain widespread credibility until the 1880s, with much research centred in France. The British Medical Association approved hypnosis as a valuable tool in 1955 and the American Medical Association followed suit in 1958.

What does it treat?

Hypnotherapy is a complementary therapy and not an alternative to seeking medical care. There are two main forms of hypnotherapy: suggestion hypnotherapy and analytical hypnotherapy.

Suggestion hypnotherapy treats problems such as giving up smoking, weight control, assertiveness, bedwetting in children, skin disorders, pre-exam nerves, and nail-biting. Analytical hypnotherapy is a combination of hypnotherapy and psychotherapy and requires between six and eight sessions. It treats more complex or chronic problems such as anxiety/panic attacks, migraine, allergies, depression, insomnia, sexual problems, obsessions and compulsions. Hypnosis can also be used for pain relief during labour and dental treatment.

A first-timer's experience
A 41-year-old male journalist

The session was held in a nice, comfortable Georgian sitting-room which is immediately relaxing. The first 40 minutes or so were spent talking. The hypnotherapist (who is also a psychotherapist) asked me about my smoking habit, when I crave cigarettes, when I had my first-ever cigarette, why I smoked, etc.

She asked me to picture myself in a social situation which is when my resolve to stop smoking breaks down. She asked me to get a visual image of that moment and look at myself from the outside. Then, she asked me to look at myself when I am not smoking and to compare how I looked and felt in each picture. In the first picture, I was skinny, fidgety and nervous with bad posture. While in the second picture, I was standing up straight, was content with myself and felt a bit like the Hollywood actor, George Clooney.

She asked me to look at the first picture and make that take up a whole screen mentally while placing the second picture in the bottom left-hand corner. She then asked me to enlarge the second picture (the one in which I wasn't smoking) and cover the first picture with it (the one in which I was smoking). She asked me to do the reverse and then the reverse of that again and again until I could no longer see the image in which I was smoking.

She then asked me to visualise myself brushing my teeth as a child, as a teenager, as a young adult, now and in ten years' time and twenty years' time. She asked me to draw a line between all these images. For me, this line curved upwards at first and then spiralled downwards off course. She asked me to straighten that line. When I mentally brought the line straight, I felt more confident and in control.

She asked me to close my eyes and think about being in a nice relaxing place. Her voice became very soothing. She continued to talk softly saying things like 'imagine yourself in a nice pool of calm, looking at the sun rippling on the surface of the water'. She talked about me going down a stairs step by step and that we were going into a deeper state of relaxation.

I felt her voice go out of my consciousness and then I heard her say, you'll wake up now. There weren't any snapping of fingers or anything like that. This part of the session took over an hour, although I didn't feel the time go by.

Afterwards, I felt very refreshed. I felt like I had a bit of mental massage and that my head had been cleared somewhat. I went out that night and I was not inclined to smoke. I listened to the tape the hypnotherapist gave me before going to sleep. I don't expect one session to cure my smoking habit, but it has given me better resolve.

An advocate's view of hypnosis to give up smoking
A 44-year-old mother of three working in the home
I had been smoking cigarettes since I was 13. I smoked 30

cigarettes a day and cigarettes were really my thing because I don't drink alcohol. I had tried giving them up with willpower (which didn't work because I have no willpower) and then using the Allen Carr method (self-suggestive techniques which work for a lot of people but not for me). So I approached hypnotherapy out of curiosity, having seen something about it on television.

When I went to the hypnotherapist, I was aware of everything that was going on although I was deeply relaxed. After the first session, I thought this hasn't worked, but in fact I have never smoked since.

The hypnotherapist asked me to throw my cigarettes in the bin after the session – which I did. I thought this is a waste because I will want a cigarette when I get to the car. I didn't. Then, I thought I will want one when I get home. I didn't.

I listened to the tape the hynotherapist gave me every morning and night for two weeks afterwards. I have had cravings but they haven't lasted for long. Each time I think of smoking or see people smoking, the idea goes out of my mind soon afterwards. I went back for a second session and for a long time I didn't believe I had given up. It was just too easy. I felt I didn't have to make an effort to give them up. I have been much more relaxed since I have given up cigarettes.

The medical view

Some general practitioners and medical specialists use hypnosis as part of their regular clinical work. There is good evidence from randomised controlled trials that hypnosis can reduce anxiety and panic disorders. Randomised trials have also shown hypnosis to be of value in asthma and irritable bowel syndrome. Hypnosis can also help in smoking cessation and with phobias such as a fear of flying. In case of abdominal pain in the absence of an identifiable physical cause, self-hypnosis was found to be of use in appropriate patients.

Choosing a practitioner

The Post-Graduate Association of the Institute of Clinical Hypnotherapy and Psychotherapy in Ireland can be contacted on tel: 021 4275785. It has 170 affiliated practising hypnotherapists. There are also up to 100 members (who have training in psychotherapy and hypnotherapy) in Neurolinguistic Programming Ireland. Tel: 01 6601578.

Members of the British Hypnotherapy Association are qualified psychotherapists. A register of members is available from 67 Upper Berkeley St, London W1H 7QX. Tel: 020 7723 4443.

Cost of treatment

A hypnotherapy session costs between €39/£30 and €105/£80.

Useful websites

www.hypnosiseire.com

Manual Lymphatic Drainage

What is it?

Experienced as a gentle form of massage, manual lymphatic drainage involves the practitioner applying gentle rhythmic pumping, scooping and stroking techniques with the hands to the skin in order to stimulate the lymphatic system. This is situated just under the skin and plays an important role in the immune system and the elimination of waste from the body. Unlike the blood, the lymphatic system has no pumps or valves to push it around the body and its organs. Instead, it must rely on movement within the body to excrete waste products.

What are its origins?

Manual lymphatic drainage was developed in France in the 1930s by a Danish massage therapist, Dr Emil Vodder. Dr Vodder's work continues to be developed and studied at the Vodder School in Austria and in many other schools throughout Germany. Manual lymphatic drainage became quickly established and accepted by conventional medicine as a treatment in France, Germany and other continental European countries. However, it is only in the last five years or so that it has gained recognition in the UK and Ireland.

What does it treat?

Manual lymphatic drainage is considered a valuable component in the treatment and control of lymphoedema (swelling of the tissues due to blockage or absence of lymph drainage channels). It is also believed to aid the healing of fractures, torn ligaments and sprains and relieves fluid congestion, swollen ankles, tired, puffy eyes, headaches and swollen legs during pregnancy. Chronic conditions such as rheumatoid arthritis and sinusitis may improve following manual lymphatic drainage. Manual lymphatic drainage is used by some healthy people as part of a detoxification programme or general health maintenance. Manual lymphatic drainage is not recommended for those with acute inflammatory or infectious conditions.

A first-timer's experience
A 50-something female secretary

Before beginning the treatment, I was asked to fill in a form with all my medical history and some details about my diet and levels of exercise. Then, I was asked to lie on my back on the treatment plinth. The therapist began with light massage strokes on my neck, under my chin and behind my ears. She moved on to the area between my neck and shoulders, using light feathery sweeping motions. I felt she had strong, sensitive hands and used good positive strokes throughout. I felt very relaxed.

She moved on to my tummy area with light brush strokes. While doing this, she asked me to practise deep abdominal breathing. She picked up that I have a particular sensitivity in this area and later showed me how to do some of the strokes myself to help relieve pain here.

Then, she gave me a facial massage, concentrating on areas of tightness she noticed across the bridge of my nose and above my eyes. I left the hour-long session feeling slightly elated and very relaxed. She advised me to drink plenty of water and not to worry if I needed to go to the toilet frequently for the rest of the day.

An advocate's view of manual lymphatic drainage for lymphoedema

A 60-year-old man who is unable to work due to severe lymphoedema
I started putting on weight about sixteen years ago and I couldn't figure out why, as I wasn't an over-eater. I just got heavier and heavier and didn't find the reason for this until three years ago on a visit to the US. While there, I discovered that I had primary lymphoedema, which is severe swelling of the body due to an accumulation of fluids.

I heard about the Vodder clinic in Austria (where special techniques have been developed to treat lymphoedema) and signed myself in for three weeks. There I had the full Vodder decongestive therapy: manual lymphatic drainage, compression therapy with bandaging, exercises and breathing. I lost five to six stones in three weeks.

Since my return from Austria, I have been having manual lymphatic drainage sessions at least once a week to stabilise my condition. Some days I feel fine and other days I'm not so good. If I get sore, I go for a treatment and feel much better afterwards. Really, I believe the treatment keeps me going at the moment.

The medical view

Lymphoedema in cancer patients can be caused by blockage of the lymphatics by a tumour or as a result of previous radiotherapy or surgery. It results in severe swelling, pain and loss of mobility. It can be treated by a combination of therapies including gentle massage which stimulates the lymphatics near the skin. This helps the accumulated fluid drain more efficiently, reduces swelling and relieves discomfort. It is a recognised form of therapy in this condition.

Choosing a practitioner

There are 14 practitioners affiliated to Manual Lymphatic

Drainage Ireland. Tel: 01 8404161. The Manual Lymphatic Drainage Association in the UK has a register of practitioners who can be contacted on tel: 01865 340385. Manual lymphatic drainage training involves one month's intensive programme at the Vodder school in Austria and two, yearly follow-up training modules. Most practitioners are also fully trained physical therapists or massage therapists.

Cost of treatment
A single treatment costs €45/£35-€52/£40.

Useful website
www.mlduk.org.uk

Massage

What is it?

Massage is by far the best known and probably the most popular complementary therapy chosen by visitors to health farms and spas. There are various techniques, strokes and degrees of hand/finger pressure used by therapists trained in different massage approaches. Relaxing background music and essential oils blended in a carrier oil are other common features.

The most common types of body massage available are Swedish massage, sports massage, shiatsu massage, aromatherapy massage and deep tissue massage. Indian head massage treats only the head, shoulders and neck areas.

What are its origins?

Massage, or the art of touch, has always existed. More formalised approaches to massage developed as part of ancient medical systems in India (the Ayurvedic system), China (traditional Chinese medicine) and Japan (also with its origins in traditional Chinese medicine).

Each approach is grounded in the philosophy of the medical system to which it belongs. Massage was also a part of Classical Greek medical studies and a regular feature at Ancient Roman baths.

Latterly, approaches inspired by these ancient systems developed in Europe. For instance, Swedish massage was developed by a nineteenth century Swedish gymnast, Per Henrik Ling. He combined ancient Chinese, Egyptian, Greek and Roman techniques with stretching exercises applied to the limbs. Sports massage, which combines pressure to the muscles through kneading, deep rubbing movements and stretching, has its origins in Russia. Many other touch therapies (including osteopathy, cranio-sacral therapy, the Bowen Technique and physical therapy) include some elements of massage.

What does it treat?

Regular massage is believed primarily to reduce stress levels. The physical effects of stress reduction include improved sleep patterns, reduced heart beat, lowered blood pressure, better blood circulation, improved immunity and energy levels.

Some forms of more vigorous massage such as Swedish or sports massage are specifically aimed at healing muscle strain or joint pain. Indian head massage is believed to relieve some forms of headaches, eye strain and sinus problems.

Massage therapy is not suitable for those with cancer, varicose veins or blood clots. Neither is it suitable for those with an acute infection (e.g. flu, fevers) or skin infections or conditions such as eczema or dermatitis.

A first-timer's experience of Swedish massage

A 36-year-old female writer

I had had one aromatherapy massage and one holistic massage some time ago, so I was interested to see if I noticed any obvious differences between these experiences and this one. The first thing I noticed was that there was no personal history taken and no questions about my health or well-being. The massage therapist said that Swedish massage was generally good for relaxation and reducing stress so the emphasis seemed to be on healthy people feeling better.

I was asked to take off my clothes down to my underwear (while the therapist left the cubicle) and lie on my back on the treatment couch. The cubicle was clean, brightly lit and painted white. The atmosphere was clinical and focussed on beauty treatments rather than a big holistic vibe with chakra charts and the like.

The therapist returned to the cubicle. She began massaging my legs and then moved to my tummy area (using light strokes only), my arms, hands, upper chest and shoulders. She then asked me to turn over onto my front. She returned to my legs and then moved on to my back. Throughout she used a sequence of massage strokes, beginning with a light stroking motion known as effleurage.

Then, she used various forms of a deeper massage which is known as petrissage. This involved kneading, knuckling and wringing actions. On my thighs and upper back, she used cupping and hacking motions. The former is noisy and feels a bit like being slapped. The latter is like a chopping action. Both of these strokes are particular to Swedish and sports massage.

The final massage stroke used was an upwards movement along either side of the spine and up along the legs and then down along the same points. This, I was told was to drain my lymph system. The treatment ended with what she called raindrops along my back – gentle finger movements up and down my back. The massage therapist didn't massage my head, face or feet during the session.

Overall, I found the treatment refreshing and relaxing. I was thirsty afterwards. I drank plenty of fluids, mainly water and tea, for the rest of the day. Unlike both my previous experiences of massage, I didn't feel at all emotional after the treatment.

An advocate's view

A 31-year-old female personal assistant

I had a car accident 12 years ago and had medical treatment at the time with inconclusive results from X-rays and bone scans. I went to an osteopath for some time to ease the pain. I had another car accident three years ago and dislocated a bone in my neck. This prevented me from going back to an osteopath.

Now, I find massage is the only thing that works for me. I get very stiff and massage relaxes me. I went for a treatment once a fortnight for quite some time. Now, I go about once every four to six weeks. I know when I need a treatment. I get a headache or my neck needs a rub out.

Initially, I was nervous about someone touching my back. But, now I find the whole ambiance distracts me from any pain I feel. It is a deep tissue massage that I get. I need the massage deep into my lower back and into my shoulders. I sleep like a baby afterwards.

The medical view

Massage is used in some disciplines of conventional medicine such as physical therapy. As a hands-on therapy, it could be seen to have a possible benefit for local injury or inflammation. However, there is no scientific evidence for its reputed health benefits. As with other complementary therapies, massage may have a placebo function through which it exerts a broad sense of well-being.

Choosing a practitioner

The Irish Massage Therapists Association has 250 members on its register. Tel: 091 589573. Members will have the letters IMTA after their name. The IMTA recognises qualifications gained through the International Training Examinations Council (ITEC) and the American Massage Therapists Association, among others.

The British Massage Therapy Council is the umbrella organisation that holds details of all accredited massage therapy schools. It is based at 17 Rymers Lane, Oxon. OX4 3JU. Tel: 01865 774123. E-mail: info@bmtc.co.uk.

Cost of treatment

A massage treatment usually costs between €39/£30 and €65/£50. Treatments in health spas and hotels may be outside this price range.

Useful website

www.bmtc.co.uk

Metamorphosis

What is it?

Metamorphosis is a hands-on therapy, applying gentle touch to the spinal reflex points of the feet, hands, head and the spine itself. Metamorphic practitioners believe that our individual experiences in the womb and at conception create the emotional patterns that carry through our lives. They believe such experiences are the roots of illness, addiction, stress, emotional problems and depression.

What are its origins?

In the 1960s, British naturopath Robert St John came up with the idea that parts of the foot – particularly the reflex areas relating to the spine – also reflected the individual's development before birth. He began to attach great importance to this prenatal period and thought that many of our physical and psychological characteristics develop during the nine-month gestation period. He decided that treatment should go back to these early patterns to remove and correct problems that begin in the first stages of life.

What does it treat?

Practitioners of metamorphosis do not diagnose or treat individual conditions but aim to treat the whole person in such a way as to promote a healthier attitude and a more sustainable way of living. The idea behind the therapy is to free us from conscious constraints we have placed on ourselves and allow a more spontaneous, natural flow to life. It originated as a therapy used to release emotional blockages in children with learning disabilities. Because it does not involve the client talking about his/her problems, people who aren't used to talking openly about their problems can find it a valuable therapy.

A first-timer's experience
A 27-year-old female writer

I went to the home of the metamorphosis practitioner and we sat down on a sofa in her living room. She asked me if I was comfortable and if I needed a glass of water or anything else. She said she wouldn't tell me what would happen in the session or what to expect.

I took off my shoes and socks and she began rubbing my feet one by one, starting with the big toe and moving on to the side of my foot and the front of my ankle. She used light, repetitive strokes that felt almost like she was washing my feet without water. She explained how the top of the big toe relates to the pre-conception period; the joint of the big toe to the point of conception and the ankle to the birthing process.

I didn't feel anything significant although I was relaxed and if anything a bit drowsy. She did the same strokes on my hands from the top of my thumb down to the joint and up my wrist. And, then on my head from the top of my crown down to my neck and around my ears, tracing a similar pattern.

She didn't ask me any questions but just chatted away about the history of metamorphosis and her own connections with it. There were points when she talked about pre-conception and the like which were too abstract for me. And, I didn't have any sense how the rubbing actions could work to unblock energy prenatally! I felt a little confused at the end of the 90-minute session. I left feeling more relaxed and as if I had just woken up. But, I went on to do my usual Friday night things feeling no different than usual.

An advocate's view

A 40-year-old full-time female student in psychology and theology

I came across metamorphosis by accident – as someone who didn't have much faith in these kind of things. In fact, I generally thought those who participated in metamorphosis and other fringe therapies were either wired to the moon or didn't have much sense. But, I changed my tune after I had a session of metamorphosis.

Directly after the session, I felt more relaxed, nothing more. But, then one week later, I started to have very vivid dreams and I began to feel completely different. It was an epochal event in my life – a strange experience. My attitude to life changed. I became more selfish, avoiding difficult situations and people rather than always giving.

My body also changed. I am an asthmatic and my asthma cleared. I started walking straighter and began to take more care of myself. I also got rid of a lot of my fears. But, still I didn't know how and why these changes came about.

That was three years ago. And, I have been back again for a few sessions since, the last of which was a year ago. I know that I will go back again if I come up against difficulties in work or relationships.

The medical view

While the concept of freeing up blocks of time to allow us to develop a healthy life is a sensible one, there is no clinical evidence to suggest that metamorphosis as a therapy brings about any specific health benefits.

Choosing a practitioner

Metamorphosis Ireland has approximately 30 qualified practitioners among its members. They can be contacted via Shiloh, Clondulane, Fermoy, Co Cork. Tel: 025 31525. E-mail: shiloh@iol.ie.

There are 20 practitioners affiliated to the Metamorphic Association, 67 Ritherdon Road, London SW17 8QE. Tel: 020 8672 5951. Metamorphosis UK can be contacted via Ann Longley, Flat D, 1a Stokenchurch St, Fulham, London SW6 3TS. Tel: 020 7384 3924.

Cost of treatment

A one-hour session costs between €39/£30 and €45/£35 (some practitioners operate a sliding scale).

Useful website

www.metamorphosis-feet.com

Nutritional Therapy

What is it?

Nutritional therapy involves the use of food and food supplements to cure and prevent disease and illness. Eating a balanced diet is so fundamental to the promotion of good health that advice on diet is usually incorporated in most treatments and therapies – both orthodox and alternative. However, nutritional therapists often take a more radical approach to diet, advising individuals to introduce completely new foods and to reduce or exclude foods which were previously a major part of their diet.

Food intolerances, food allergies and long-term toxic reactions to certain foods are identified and treated. Food supplements may also be prescribed to correct any mineral and vitamin imbalances detected. Nutritional therapists usually also stress the value of eating fresh, organic food and drinking natural spring water.

What are its origins?

Nutritional therapy could be said to be one of the oldest therapies, as the idea that food is medicine has been around since Ancient Greece. Yet, in another way, it has only recently gained credence as a therapy in itself.

Although scientific discoveries of minerals and vitamins didn't occur until the early twentieth century, many systems of medicine including the Ayurvedic system in India and traditional Chinese medicine always included food or diet therapy as an important part of overall healthy living.

Polish scientist Casimir Funk is credited with the discovery of vitamins. The study of minerals in food began in the 1940s. Since then, research into foods rich in vitamins and minerals and their importance for certain illnesses has grown hugely.

What does it treat?

Nutritional therapy can treat a wide variety of ailments including migraine, hay fever, food allergies, eczema, asthma, inflammatory diseases such as osteoarthritis, fatigue, ME, fluid retention, irritable bowel syndrome and other digestive disorders.

A first-timer's experience

A 30-year-old female selling agent

I work for myself and I realised recently that I was always tired and stressed out. Even though I get about eight or nine hours sleep at night, I would wake up feeling tired and this feeling would hang over me all day. I heard of a nutritional therapist through word of mouth and decided to go to her.

She began by asking me about my medical history, my family's medical history, my lifestyle, my levels of exercise and my diet. Then, she did a series of kinesiology tests. [Kinesiology testing is used by various alternative and complementary practitioners as a diagnostic method. By testing the strength of various muscles in the body, the level of functioning of organs, digestive system, glands, bones and circulation is calculated.] While she was doing this, I was lying on a plinth. It was very relaxing.

Following these tests, she said I was only using about 50 per cent of my brain. She recommended that I have 20 minutes exercise a day and 20 minutes sunlight a day. She also suggested that I drink still mineral water and that I give up alcohol for a while to see how my body would react. She said I should stay away from foods containing yeast and sugar and eat more fresh vegetables, preferably organic. She also prescribed a list of supplements which I could try.

After the hour-long consultation, I felt that making the changes to my diet would require a big effort. However, I was relieved to have found a way that would help me stop feeling I needed to sleep all the time.

An advocate's view of nutritional therapy and ME
A 53-year-old female healer

I had been diagnosed with ME and later developed septicaemia in my foot and an ulcer in my leg. I had received orthodox treatment for these conditions but I felt I was still very unwell. This is when I went to a nutritional therapist.

She prescribed some homeopathic remedies and some flower remedies. I had a largely organic diet of grains (brown rice and millet), which have a lot of healing properties, and organic vegetables. I avoided dairy foods and products with wheat and sugar. I started taking quite a lot of nutritional supplements which included immune boosters such as echinacea, garlic, vitamin C and Udos oils and greens. I meditated and walked regularly, though it was hard initially because of the pain in my foot. Now, one and a half years later, my leg has healed. I feel so well. I rarely have any tiredness. I still take some supplements. When I stray from my diet and supplements, I get a nudge reminding me to come back to it. All is well.

The medical view

It can be difficult to differentiate between conventional and complementary nutritional therapies. The evidence for unconventional nutritional interventions is generally either non-existent or negative. There has been no rigorous research on individualised nutritional therapies.

Choosing a practitioner

Members of the British Association of Nutritional Therapists in the UK and Ireland can be contacted via 27 Old Gloucester St, London WC1 3XX. Tel: 0870 6061284 (for phoning from the UK only).

Members of the Register of Nutritional Therapists can be contacted on email: pennywoolley@talk21.com.

Cost of treatment

Consultations cost from €39/£30 per visit.

Useful websites

www.bant.org.uk

Osteopathy

What is it?

Osteopathy involves the gentle manipulation of the joints and spinal vertebrae coupled with massage and stretching of the muscles and ligaments. Osteopaths believe that the correct functioning of our musculo-skeletal system has a profound influence on the workings of our internal organs and on our general health. They assert that the mechanics of the body can be distorted by bad posture, injury and stress leading to pain and strain. This can in turn affect breathing, blood circulation and digestion. Equally, internal problems can lead to muscular pain, as our body structure tries to compensate for the internal imbalance.

Cranial osteopathy is a more recently developed form of osteopathy which concerns itself with the gentle manipulation of the head, spine and sacrum in order to restore the free flow of cranial fluid.

What are its origins?

The word 'osteopathy' is a combination of the Greek *osteon* meaning bone and *pathos* meaning pain or suffering. Its founder, Andrew Taylor Still (1828-1917) trained as a doctor, but became disillusioned with medicine and the prescription of the often dangerous drugs of his day. He became convinced that many illnesses arise when part of the body's structure becomes out of alignment. He developed a system of medicine designed to adjust the body's structure to enable it to function well enough to heal itself and deal with disease. He established the first school of osteopathy in Kirksville, Missouri, USA, in 1892.

What does it treat?

Osteopathy is considered a very good therapy for back, neck and shoulder pain and sports injuries. It is also considered to be valuable for occupational strain in the joints and muscles. Conditions such as asthma, premenstrual tension and migraine are also believed to respond well to osteopathy, as is backache during pregnancy.

Osteopathy is not recommended for those with cancer of the bone or joint. Neither is it a suitable treatment for fractures. However, it can treat weakness resulting from a fracture, once the fracture has been medically treated.

Cranial osteopathy is considered valuable for babies with colic, older children with behavioural problems and adults with stress-related illnesses. See also Cranio-sacral therapy.

A first-timer's experience

A 35-year-old female journalist

I had some idea what osteopathy was about so I was prepared for some gentle physical manipulation of my spine. The session began with a discussion about any particular areas of physical weakness or pain in my body, in my case the joints and muscles of my arms. As I lay on the treatment couch, the osteopath moved my arms from the elbow joints and worked into any tightness in the muscle. This felt comforting and relieved some of the pain I had felt in the area.

Then, while asking questions about my general health, lifestyle and if I had any accidents or injuries, he began working on my neck, extending it upwards off my back with firm yet gentle movements of his hands. This left the impression that my neck should perhaps be longer than it usually is. Following this, he held my head and made clicking sounds as he moved my neck from one side to the other.

Later, he asked me to cross my arms over my chest and moved down my back with his hands, checking the vertebrae and musculature of my spine. He also checked the position of my pelvis. After this, he checked my sitting and standing postures.

Following the 40-minute session, he assessed my overall condition and said that I would benefit from some more treatments. He also gave me some advice on easing the strain on my body while I work. Things like using a wrist rest in front of my keyboard and using a headset while on the telephone. I left feeling uplifted and brighter, keen to make the ergonomic changes as soon as possible.

An advocate's view of osteopathy for whiplash

A 23-year-old woman working in sales and marketing

I was in a car crash three and a half years ago and I suffered a lot of muscle damage to my back, neck and shoulders. I attended a physiotherapist regularly for about eight months without feeling that my muscles loosened up much at all. The physiotherapist suggested that I give up treatment for a while to allow some self-healing. Meanwhile, I continued to take anti-inflammatory painkillers.

After another couple of months, I went to an osteopath on the recommendation of my physiotherapist. When, I first attended the osteopath, he was surprised to find I had such restricted movement. I couldn't turn my head very far from side to side or move my chin up and down to any great extent.

For about three months, I went to the osteopath two or three times a week. After each session, I felt my neck was a lot looser for a few days and then it would tighten up again. However, within a few months, I began to notice huge changes. I could turn my head further from side to side. Now, over two years later, I am still attending my osteopath every three or four weeks. I can move my head about 50 per cent to one side and about 70 per cent to the other side. I feel I will not be completely better until I can move my head completely from side to side. However, I do not suffer any pain at all unless I have had a particularly stressful day.

The medical view
Osteopathy is accepted as a legitimate medical treatment by a substantial number of conventional doctors. The Royal College of General Practitioners include osteopathy in their recommendations for physical therapy in the treatment of persisting uncomplicated back pain. There is considerable evidence from randomised controlled trials of the effectiveness of osteopathy for back and neck pain. The side effects include discomfort at the site of manipulation, headache and fatigue. Most of these complaints resolve within 24 hours. Estimates of spinal cord injury following forceful manipulation range from one patient in 20,000 to one patient in a million.

Choosing a practitioner
There are 100 osteopaths registered with the Irish Osteopathic Association, 10 Winton Avenue, Rathgar, Dublin 6. Tel: 01 2695281/091 589417. E-mail: karlp@iol.ie.

There are approximately 2,500 osteopaths registered with the General Osteopathic Council, Osteopathy House, 176 Tower Bridge Road, London SE1 3LU. Tel: 020 7357 6655. E-mail: info@osteopathy.org.uk.

Registered osteopaths in Ireland will often have the letters MIOA after their name. Also osteopaths in Britain and Ireland will have

DO (Diploma in osteopathy) or BSc Ost. Med/Ost. or perhaps MSc.

Cost of treatment

Treatments cost from €32/£25 to €45/£35 (for 20 and 30 minutes). The first visit may cost from €39/£30 to €52/£40 and lasts between 30 and 45 minutes. In Ireland, BUPA offer €20/£15 towards each osteopathic treatment by members of the IOA, while VHI offer €20/£15 towards osteopathic treatments carried out by GPs. In the UK, BUPA and PPP offer reductions for osteopathic treatments. Osteopathy is also available on the NHS through GP referral.

Useful website

www.osteopathy.org.uk

Physical Therapy

What is it?
Physical therapy is a form of treatment that combines deep tissue massage with joint movement. Its aim is to restore joint mobility and ease muscular tension. As with massage therapy, the hands-on method also improves blood circulation and removes toxins from the body.

What are its origins?
The nineteenth-century Swedish gymnast, Per Henrik Ling, is considered the originator of both Swedish massage and physical therapy. He combined a series of active and passive movements of the joints with massage in his treatment approach. After initial opposition in medical circles, the techniques became accepted and Dutch physician Johann Mezger is given credit for introducing massage as a form of medical treatment.

Further research in the 1940s and 1950s by orthopaedic surgeon James Henry Cyriax emphasised the fact that pain could be caused by soft-tissue dysfunction. This became the foundation of soft-tissue manipulation today. Schools of physical therapy were established in the US, the UK and Ireland in the 1980s.

What does it treat?
Designed to treat disorders of the musculo-skeletal system,

physical therapy is effective for back and neck conditions, sports injuries including joint strains and sprains, tennis and golfer's elbow, tension headaches, postural aches and pains, whiplash, fibrositis (inflammation of fibrous tissue) and arthritis. Long-standing medical complaints may require medical diagnosis before treatment can begin.

A first-timer's experience
A 51-year-old mother of four
I went to the physical therapist with pain in my knees which I have had for some time. Before beginning the treatment, she asked me if I was on any medication. She also asked about my lifestyle and hobbies with the view to finding out when my knees hurt most.

She asked me to stand and felt under my arches, my legs and my knees. Then, she asked me to lie down and moved my legs from side to side to see if there was any ligament damage. She also stretched my legs up towards the ceiling, noting that I had good movement in my legs. She then felt up along my legs from the knee to the thigh, noting that the muscle was tighter and more knotted on the outside of my legs.

Following this, she did some deep massage into the outer sides of my legs to ease the muscle out. Although it wasn't painful as such, I could feel a strong pressure into my legs, which left them feeling tingly. She asked me to turn over on my stomach and worked into the back side of my legs. Then, she moved my legs backwards towards my bottom. I felt I had more mobility after the treatment and less of the dull pain in my knees.

I was however a bit surprised that the therapist didn't look at my spine or other areas of my body to check my overall posture. She told me to drink plenty of water after the treatment.

An advocate's view of physical therapy for tennis elbow

A 24-year-old male sales executive

I got a lot of pain around my elbow and into my elbow joint last February. I was playing quite a bit of tennis and it is the busiest time of the year for us at work so I was using the computer a lot. I ignored the pain for a while and it got worse. Then, I went to my GP who prescribed anti-inflammatories. These gave me slight relief over the next three weeks or so. But, then through someone in the club, I heard about physical therapy and made an appointment to see a physical therapist. I had five treatments in all.

After an initial assessment, the therapist concluded the problem derived as much from my work on the computer as from playing tennis. At each session, she did deep tissue massage work around the area of pain and also in my neck. I had a lingering pain in my neck from turning my head sideways towards the computer. I experienced a huge reduction in pain between the first and second sessions. Then, over the following three weeks with one session a week, the pain eased completely. I believe now that working into the area which was tight cured the pain.

I have been given stretching exercises to do every day which I do about three or four times a week. Initially, I used ice on the area every morning to bring down any inflammation, but I don't need to do that anymore. I can play tennis now without wincing with pain and type away on the computer without any problems.

The medical view

Per Henrik Ling believed massage could bring about healing by improving circulation. Complementary therapists have adapted Ling's theories so as to place a greater emphasis on the psychological benefits of treatment. Massage therapists generally have moved away from loosening stiff joints and improving blood flow.

Physical-therapy techniques do emphasise the stretching of

muscles and joints and there is some evidence to suggest the effectiveness of massage in improving circulation and decreasing muscle tension. There is no reliable data to link these changes with clinical benefits such as increased mobility or improved athletic performance.

Choosing a practitioner
There are approximately 85 physical therapists registered with the Irish Association of Physical Therapists. Tel: 01 2835566. E-mail: iapt@clubi.ie. All registered physical therapists have completed a three-year diploma course in physical therapy.

Cost of treatment
Each treatment costs between €32/£25 and €45/£35 per 45-minute session.

Useful website
www.iptas.com

Rebirthing

What is it?

Rebirthing is a breathing technique used principally as a psychotherapeutic tool to gain access to blocked experiences and emotions. It involves the individual practising a form of shallow breathing under the guidance of the rebirthing therapist. The ideology behind rebirthing is that the breathing technique allows the individual to enter past painful experiences (in a faster way than by 'talk therapy' alone) and go through them in a safe, protected therapeutic situation so as to free him/herself of emotional, physical or mental blockages. The therapy is called rebirthing because some clients experience something akin to their birth experience during the treatment.

What are its origins?

The roots of rebirthing can be found in ancient yoga traditions in India and in the Chinese qi gong system of exercises. In its present form, rebirthing was developed in the United States in the late 1960s and early 1970s by business consultant Leonard Orr. Together with medical nurse Sondra Ray, he developed rebirther training courses. The therapy was called rebirthing because the first experience of the pioneers of the therapy (and that of many first-timers) was a memory of their birth.

Throughout the 1980s and 1990s, various approaches to

rebirthing developed in Europe, the United States, Australia and Russia. In 1994, they came together to form the International Breathwork Foundation. Through the work of the IBF, rebirthing slowly began to gain acceptance as a legitimate tool of psychotherapy.

What does it treat?

Rebirthing is a complementary therapy within the domain of psychotherapy. It is deemed useful for depression, relationship difficulties, job problems, stress, panic attacks, anxiety, phobias and other psychological problems.

It is not suitable for those with psychotic disorders such as schizophrenia, manic depression or paranoia. Neither is it appropriate for people in crisis who have not had a history of self-development to build on.

A first-timer's experience

A 38-year-old female writer

The therapist began by talking about what rebirthing involved and how more emphasis should be on the in breath than the out breath. She explained how we store our emotions in the area between our upper lungs and our collar bone. She warned me that certain things might happen: that I might relive my birth experience; that I might go into another memory or emotion; that I might feel some localised physical pain or movement or energy in my body and that I probably would go into some kind of non-ordinary state of consciousness. The breathing had to be quite quick and without pause, she said as she demonstrated it to me. She also said that it is useful to think of one particular issue or problem before beginning. Then, we began.

I spent a short time talking to her about the issue I would bring to the session. Then, I lay on the bed. She sat beside me and began to do the shallow breathing so that I might get into the correct rhythm. Soon, I began to feel quite uncomfortable: my chest started burning and I had pins and needles in my hands and feet. I became resistant to the breathing, as I felt I wasn't getting enough air in and didn't have enough time to get the breath out fully. I began to breathe very rapidly and the therapist said just keep breathing.

After complaining a bit and alternating nose breathing with mouth breathing, the pins and needles began to spread all over my body. I also began to feel quite dizzy. I felt like my whole body and head were being flattened in a vice-like grip (this was interesting I thought because my birth had been a forceps delivery). My forearms and hands also locked in position. I felt quite distressed. I had an earache, a pain in my back and I began to get a bit fed up of the whole thing. I asked the therapist why I was clenching like that and she said that maybe there was something I was holding onto.

She asked me what I saw and I saw a man in a white coat with a tweezers in his hand. I laughed and said, so this is the doctor who delivered me. But then I saw a coffin and I felt like I was being placed in this coffin and put down into the ground. I found this very upsetting and began to cry. I began to think about my mother's first baby who died. I got very upset thinking about this baby and realised I had a lot of unexpressed grief around this. I also realised that I was hanging on to some of my mother's unexpressed grief about this baby's death. I started to breathe more slowly and I began to feel my body relax and my hands unclench.

We talked about my experience. The therapist said that I don't have to be responsible for my mother's grief and she suggested I say this to myself on a regular basis. I felt very light-headed and peculiar after the two-hour session. I got up and we sat and talked over a cup of tea. I felt very drained and tired but also I had a sense of release having cried.

As an adult, you don't often get the space to have a good cry. I had felt safe and supported throughout the session. I think that rebirthing is a powerful technique, but if used in the wrong hands the experience could be a rather dark one.

An advocate's view of rebirthing and depression

A 41-year-old health practitioner working in private practice

My lifestyle appeared excellent – my husband and I both had full-time, well-paid jobs, three holidays a year and a lovely house. But, I wasn't happy. I didn't know what I wanted in life or where I was going. I gave up my job and became self-employed, but I still couldn't cope. I went to my GP who referred me to a psychiatrist who started talking about ECT and the like, which just wasn't for me. I had a panic attack which was a point of crisis for me. I decided to take a complete break. I went abroad for three months to contemplate things.

I had tried rebirthing before I left with little gain. But while I was abroad, I did some more rebirthing sessions that led to a breakthrough for me. In my family of origin, I am the youngest and soaked up all the emotional problems in the family. This had really affected me and made me very unhappy. These problems had also transferred into my other close relationships.

Rebirthing allowed me to realise these things and change my role within my family of origin. It also gave me the clarity of thought that allowed me to sit down and work things out. I began to realise that I had barely scratched the surface of my own potential. When you are doing a rebirthing session, you connect with something deep inside you. I needed to do this. What started off as a psychotherapeutic intervention has become something more spiritual. It's the simplicity of rebirthing which really appeals to me: there's nothing more to it than using the breathing techniques and having the willingness to do so with the support of a rebirther.

The medical view

I am not aware of clinical evidence to support its effectiveness in any medical conditions.

Choosing a practitioner

There are approximately 50 practitioners of rebirthing in Ireland, trained in various schools. The Rebirthing Association of Ireland can be contacted on tel: 01 4533166.

The British Rebirthing Society can be contacted via Clare Gabriel, 59b Panmure Close, Highbury, London N1 1AG. Tel: 020 7704 8803. E-mail: claregabriel@globalpeaceuk.com.

Cost of treatment

A rebirthing session of two to two and a half hours costs between €39/£30 and €130/£100.

Useful websites

www.ibfnetwork.org
www.i-breathe.com

Reflexology

What is it?

Reflexology is based on the principle that there are reflex points in the hands and feet which correspond to the glands, organs and other parts of the body. By applying pressure to specific areas on the feet or hands with the thumbs and fingers, reflexologists seek to alleviate or treat a range of conditions.

Each reflex point reflects the state of the body part or organ by its feel and condition, and practitioners can sometimes detect weaknesses before they start to cause problems. The left foot represents the left side of the body and the right foot represents the right side. Most practising reflexologists prefer to work with feet as they are larger and more sensitive than hands.

What are its origins?

Reflexology originated in China over five thousand year ago as a form of pressure therapy. The Ancient Egyptians also used a form of reflexology, as did many African tribes and Native American Indians. It was not until the early twentieth century that the therapy was introduced into the West by American ear, nose and throat consultant Dr William Fitzgerald. He devised a method called Zone Therapy that involved the use of healing pressure on various points within ten zones along the body.

American physiotherapist Eunice Ingham adapted Fitzgerald's

therapy by treating the body through pressure applied only to the feet. She mapped out areas of the feet that when stimulated by pressure were likely to have a therapeutic effect. Reflexology was introduced to the UK in the 1960s by a student of Ingham's, Doreen Bayly.

What does it treat?

Reflexology is not a substitute for medical care and reflexologists do not diagnose conditions. As a complementary therapy, it is deemed a valued treatment for migraine, high blood pressure, back and neck pain, sinus and menstrual problems, irritable bowel syndrome and other stress-related ailments. It is also considered useful in preventative healthcare, as it brings about deep relaxation, improves blood circulation and clears the body of toxins and impurities.

Some reflexologists will not treat those with acute infections, heart disease, osteoporosis, diabetes or epilepsy. Anyone who has had hip or knee replacements should not have reflexology until the area is completely healed. It has been claimed that having reflexology during pregnancy can significantly reduce the length of labour.

A first-timer's experience

A 31-year-old female hat designer

I have a sensitive scar on the top of my left foot so I was a little nervous in case the treatment might cause pain to this area. After a few questions about my health (such as if I had had any operations, if I was pregnant or using an intrauterine devise as a contraceptive) and reassurance that she wouldn't touch my scar, the reflexologist asked me to take off my shoes and socks and lie down on her treatment couch.

I thought the treatment would feel like a foot massage but it was much more intensive than any foot massage I've had. She worked on each foot separately, starting with the left and using gentle strokes followed by firmer pressure and some squeezing actions on my toes. It was very relaxing and there was gentle music playing in the background.

The reflexologist dealt comprehensively with the sides, sole and top of each foot and every part of all my toes. At certain points, I squirmed with pain. Following the treatment, she referred back to the points when it hurt and asked me about specific illnesses or ailments, some of which I had experienced. She explained that the purpose of the first treatment was to release all toxins through the feet. More specific problems would take further treatment to heal. She also advised me to drink plenty of water afterwards. I was completely relaxed and a bit drowsy after the treatment which lasted about eighty minutes.

An advocate's view of reflexology and neck pain
A 46-year-old mother working in the home
I had a cyst on my ear five years ago and three weeks after surgery I went for my first reflexology treatment. I also had facial paralysis at this time and days after my first reflexology treatment, I felt the nerves coming back into my face. At that time, I had weekly treatments for six weeks which brought me fully back to normal.

At the moment, I am attending my reflexologist for a pain in my neck so I go about once a fortnight. I find that my neck is becoming much looser and not at all as stiff. My reflexologist deals specifically with an area on my foot that is linked to my neck. When my neck is better, I will continue to go for treatments about once a month as part of a health maintenance programme.

I love it. It is so relaxing. The actions don't tickle your feet. They are quite firm. I believe reflexology deals directly with different parts of the body because the feet are a map of the body. It really keeps the balance right for me.

The medical view

There are no published research studies on the effectiveness of reflexology as a medical treatment. A 1994 study of the use of complementary medicine by cancer patients attending a London hospital oncology unit showed reflexology was one of the least used therapies. Reflexology is likely to have beneficial psychological effects. There is no evidence of any side effects or harm emanating from reflexology.

Choosing a practitioner

There are approximately 1,000 practising reflexologists in Ireland.

The Irish Reflexologists Institute is the largest association of reflexologists with approximately 700 members, all of whom have 70 hours of training and 60 reported treatments. Tel: 028 91462657.

There are 6,500 members in the Association of Reflexologists, 27 Old Gloucester St, London WC1N 3XX. Tel: 0870 5673320 (for phoning from the UK only). E-mail: aor@reflexology.org. All members must have six to nine months training (accredited courses have 100 contact teaching hours and 60 treatments before certificate and six detailed case studies). Once in professional practice for one year, members of the Association of Reflexologists can use MAR after their name.

Cost of treatment

Treatment costs ranges from €26/£20 to €39/£30.

Useful websites

www.reflexology.ie
www.aor.org.uk

Reiki

What is it?
Reiki (pronounced ray-kee) is a hands-on therapy which is believed to promote the flow of energy through the body. Practitioners maintain that by using a specific series of hand positions on various points on the individual client, that person will draw energy from the practitioner's hands to where it is needed in his/her body. Considered an easy to learn art or technique, lay people can learn how to use reiki on themselves and their families. There is however a longer training and initiation period for those who wish to become reiki masters or teachers.

What are its origins?
Reiki is a Japanese word which is formed from the word *rei* (universal) and *ki* (life energy). It has its roots in ancient Tibetan Buddhist healing and was practised by ancient Tibetans, Chinese, Egyptians and Japanese.

The Usui system is the form of reiki most widely practised in the West. It was developed in the mid 1800s by Dr Mikao Usui, a Japanese Christian theologian. Through his studies, Dr Usui rediscovered the ancient techniques and spent his life practising and teaching his method of natural healing. Reiki was brought to the West by a female practitioner, Hawaio Takata, in the 1960s.

What does it treat?

Reiki is a complementary therapy and not an alternative to orthodox medical treatment. Its benefits are seen to be in helping people to relax and de-stress themselves. Sufferers of arthritis, back pain, depression and other stress-related disorders have found relief with reiki. It is also used by some practitioners as an after-care therapy with cancer patients.

Reiki is not given to anyone who has just fractured a limb and has not had medical treatment. It can also be uncomfortable to receive if the individual is suffering from a high fever. Inflamed skin is not touched by a reiki practitioner. According to its practitioners, reiki can be administered from a distance.

A first-timer's experience

A 30-year-old female fashion designer

The reiki master began by telling me all about reiki and asked me my age; what I did for a living; if I had had any operations, and if I was on any medication. She then asked me to lie down on her plinth with two pillows under my head and two pillows under my knees. (Prior to the session, I had been advised to wear loose, comfortable clothing.)

She began by placing both her hands over my eyes for about five minutes. Her hands began to feel very hot while there. Then, she placed her hands on the top of my head, the back of my head and on my temples. Each time, she left them there for five minutes or more. Then, she moved on to my chest, lower ribs, stomach, abdomen, again leaving her hands in each place for five minutes or so.

I had my eyes closed during this time and I felt like I was in a trance. I found myself daydreaming about things I had to do, but rather than getting stressed about them, they came into my head and just floated away again. During this time, my stomach started gurgling and later I began to pass wind. This was a little embarrassing, but the reiki practitioner said not to worry, that this was normal.

She asked me to turn over and began using the same hand positions on my shoulders, my upper back, my lower back and my bottom. During all this time, I believe I felt more relaxed than I have ever felt. I had no concept of time, but the whole session took about one and a half hours. When it was complete, I felt quite light-headed. She asked me if I suffered a lot from constipation which I do. She said that she had felt this problem in my body. She also said that it was related to there being a lot of things going on for me about which I found difficulty expressing my views and feelings. After the session, I felt very tearful. Then, I started to laugh. Later, that evening, I felt fine – just completely tired.

An advocate's view of reiki for feelings of dissatisfaction with life

A 53-year-old businessman

I first heard of reiki a long time ago. However, it was four years ago when I had my first treatments (four in a row, which is the recommended number to begin with). At that time, I wasn't content with my life and I didn't know why. Basically, if you are open to reiki, it makes you confront areas in your life. And it made me confront personal and work issues instead of burying them.

I began to think about things such as that we are all individually responsible for our own lives and the direction they take. Reiki helped me get rid of anger, resentment and blame I had towards other people. I can honestly say that these emotions no longer exist in my life. And instead of trying to lead my life through other people, I became more content with my own company. It also made me realise that the past is gone. We are living for now and the future is a dream which may never come true. So, I don't live in fear of the future anymore.

Reiki has also made me better at my job and more focussed. Instead of compromising on issues, now if I think I am correct, nobody will change my view. I have a reiki treatment irregularly now – whenever I need one. Basically, it's whenever my head becomes too cluttered with things which are not important. Reiki just seems to get rid of that clutter.

The medical view

Reiki therapy may help patients by offering general relaxation. This therapy does not lend itself to research in clinical medicine trials. Any claims that it treats specific conditions should be viewed with caution.

Choosing a practitioner

There are currently 10 practitioners of reiki who have been assessed and approved to give reiki treatments to members of the public by the Reiki Association of Ireland. Tel: 021 371058. There are many more practitioners who have varying levels of training, some of whom use reiki combined with other therapies. As with other therapies, clients should be cautious about receiving reiki from practitioners not recommended by the Reiki associations.

The Reiki Association of Great Britain has a list of 44 members who give Reiki treatments professionally. Details from Julie Prescott-Rogers, 8 Windmill Close, Buerton, Crewe CW3 ODF. Tel: 01270 812829. E-mail: reikiassoc-admin@compuserve.com.

Cost of treatment

A single reiki session costs between €26/£20 and €52/£40.

Useful websites

www.reikiassocation.org.uk
www.reiki.org

Shiatsu

What is it?

Shiatsu means finger pressure in Japanese. It involves the application of pressure from the thumbs, palms of the hands and sometimes elbows and knees to specifically designated points (*tsubos*) along the meridians (energy pathways as defined by traditional Chinese medicine) of the body.

An important part of the consultation is *hara* diagnosis, which involves the practitioner placing the palm of one hand on the abdomen and the other hand feeling the area with the tips of the fingers. This process tells the practitioner which meridians should be worked on. Some stretching and holding techniques may also be incorporated into the treatment.

Like acupuncturists, shiatsu practitioners believe that illness or dysfunction results from blockage, under-activity or over-activity in the energy pathways which are linked to the organs and systems of the body.

What are its origins?

Shiatsu is often described as acupuncture without needles. Both acupuncture and shiatsu have their origins in traditional Chinese medicine. Shiatsu in its present form was revived in Japan in the early twentieth century by Tokujiro Namikoshi.

Schools of shiatsu opened throughout the Western world in the 1980s and 1990s. Various styles of shiatsu have developed over the last forty years. The main ones are Zen shiatsu, Oha shiatsu, Nippon, Macrobiotic shiatsu and Five Elements shiatsu.

What does it treat?

As with virtually all alternative therapies, shiatsu treats the whole person (mind, body and spirit) and seeks out the fundamental cause of the problem, rather than solely concentrating on local symptoms. It is however deemed a valuable treatment for back pain, shoulder tension, headaches, some skin and digestive conditions, anxiety and insomnia. It can also be used alongside allopathic medicine to enhance recovery from serious illnesses.

The treatment is given through the clothes, while the patient lies on a soft mat on the floor. Some people become so relaxed that they enter a deeper level of consciousness during a shiatsu session.

Shiatsu is not recommended for those with acute illnesses with fever. Practitioners will work more sensitively with clients with osteoporosis, inflamed joints, varicose veins, wounds or fractures and pregnant women.

A first-timer's experience
A 37-year-old female writer

Upon making the appointment, I was advised to wear loose, comfortable clothing and to have eaten at least one and a half hours before the treatment. The first 20 minutes of the session was spent answering questions about the specific reason for coming for treatment (lower back pain, in my case), my lifestyle, past illnesses, job satisfaction, diet, exercise and how I expressed myself creatively. I felt the practitioner was very thorough and in no rush through these questions. He was relaxed, friendly and attentive to my answers.

Then, to my surprise I was asked to lie on my back on a mat on the floor (I expected a plinth of some sort). He picked up my right arm and stretched it out, putting pressure at certain points. Then, he put his hand on my stomach and putting deep pressure on it, rolled it back and forth like a piece of pastry. This felt a little uncomfortable.

He lifted my legs up and balancing them on his chest, pushed my legs down so that my knees were bent into my chest with the soles of my feet remaining on his chest. This gave my spine a really good stretch. Later he moved behind my head, turning my neck from side to side, whilst putting pressure on the area where my skull meets my neck.

This felt firm, yet very relaxing and pleasant. As time went on, I began to feel deeply relaxed and almost drifting in and out of sleep. At one point, the shiatsu practitioner stood over me and put his hands into the curve of my back, lifting me upwards. This felt nice, although I wondered how high he would lift my body. He also did some work on my arms and wrists and I was surprised at how sore they were.

At another point, he pushed my shoulders back towards the floor. Then, I was asked to turn onto my tummy. Once there, he gave me another strong leg stretch and bent my knees right back into my buttocks. He worked all over my spine with the flat part of his hands and his fingers. I felt he was really concentrating throughout and interacting with me on quite a profound level.

At the end of the one-and-a-half hour session, he left me lying down for a while and then slowly invited me back to a sitting position, after I had first walked around for a bit. He said I would benefit from a few more sessions if the pain returned to my lower back. He also recommended the Alexander Technique to improve my posture and showed me a point on my calf to press to help me cope with the pain in my lower back. I felt some tenderness in this area after the session.

An advocate's view of shiatsu for back pain
A 33-year-old female administrator

A year and a half ago, when I developed a recurring pain in my lower back, I opted for shiatsu as a means of treatment. Having watched my father suffer from a degenerative disc disease for many years and witnessed the scale of physical and chemical intervention prescribed by Western medicine and its debatable success, I was anxious not to launch myself down a similar path.

Now, a year and some months later, I have been for over 40 shiatsu sessions. Within three months of treatment, I wasn't experiencing the same level of pain from my back. I still look forward to each session before I go and so far, I have never walked out of a treatment having had the same experience twice. There have been sessions during and after which I have experienced moments of extraordinary physical well-being and others where it has been hard to lie still on the mat for the whole session.

Some sessions have been relaxing and others challenging and even tiring. Overall, my experience of shiatsu has been profoundly healing. My back is much stronger but, more than anything, I have come to realise in my physical being, the interconnectedness between mind and body. I have learned to realise that each breath I take brings new life to my body and that sometimes when life gets too hectic, that to just keep breathing in and out is enough of an achievement.

The medical view
There are no clinical trials on the medical effects of shiatsu. However, as the therapy uses pressure on acupuncture points, it is reasonable to expect it to be more effective in relieving pain than a

'sham' technique. Its proponents emphasise its broad health improving benefits; these are far too broad to ever lend themselves to scientific analysis.

Choosing a practitioner
There are 25 practitioners registered with the Shiatsu Association of Ireland, which can be contacted at PO Box 7683, Malahide, Co. Dublin. Tel: 01 2604669.

The Shiatsu Society UK has about 2,000 members. They can be contacted via their offices at Eastlands Court, St Peters Road, Rugby, CV21 3QP. Tel: 01788 555051. E-mail: admin@shiatsu.org. Professional training varies from three to four years.

Cost of treatment
Individual treatments cost €26/£20 to €45/£35 per one-hour session (the first treatment lasts one and a half hours).

Useful websites
www.shiatsuireland.com
www.shiatsu.org

Spiritual Healing

What is it?
Spiritual healing involves the therapist connecting with the spiritual energy flowing in and around the individual client and adjusting it as a means towards resolving underlying physical, emotional, mental or indeed spiritual stress. It is based on the principle that a lot of sickness and disease has its roots in spiritual malaise.

Spiritual healers use techniques such as the laying on of hands, connecting psychically with the individual and reading and working with auras. Each person is believed to be surrounded by an area of light that connects with a universal field of spiritual energy. The light is believed to be composed of seven different coloured rays, each associated with particular organs and emotions.

The tools used by spiritual healers vary, but generally speaking pendulums, crystals, tarot cards, semiprecious stones and aura soma bottles are used. Aura soma bottles are clear glass bottles of crystal-clear oils, plant extracts and essences used to revitalise and rebalance the human aura.

What are its origins?
Spiritual healing has been practised in various forms since time began. The techniques and tools may vary between practitioners and across different cultures, but the aim is the same – to channel healing energy towards the person who needs it.

What does it treat?

Spiritual healers claim some success in the relief of back pain, sciatica, depression, stress-related disorders and emotional traumas. Unlike faith healing, spiritual healing is claimed to take place without the patient having faith in the healer or the healing process.

A first-timer's experience

A 50-year-old mother of four

First off, I was surprised that the healer was young and beautiful. I had expected someone broody, dark and intense. Also, she wasn't at all invasive and clearly inhabited her own space. She began by asking me to select a bottle from a choice of coloured bottles (aura soma bottles) and a stone from a group of semiprecious stones and crystals. I selected a blue bottle. Then, I selected a turquoise stone which I held in my left hand throughout the whole session. Then, she asked me to lie on the plinth and handed me a clear quartz crystal to hold in my right hand.

She moved around my whole body, holding her hands at a distance from my body as she moved. Then, she did some laying on of hands. She held my head and then put her hands under my neck, on my knees and on my hips. I have been in a lot of pain with my neck and back in the last few weeks, which I explained to her. And, when she placed her hands on my left hip, I felt a great heat (I am a sceptic about these things but I did feel heat).

Then, she asked me to turn over onto my front and she laid her hands at the same points on my back. Again, when she laid her hands on the area around my lungs, I felt an intense heat.

We spoke about my family, particularly my mother who died two years ago. She said some things about my mother and I that made some sense, but other things which didn't seem significant.

She also used a pendulum to figure out what I am doing which is bad for my health. She then recommended I stop doing the front crawl when swimming and to do the breast stroke instead. I would be very sceptical about this sort of advice, but as a regular swimmer I will give it a go for a week or two. She also asked me to choose one of the coloured bottles (aura soma bottles, again) and I chose gold. She said this was significant because it related to my torso from where my physical pain originated. I bought one of these gold bottles to rub the contents of which around my abdomen and back.

Immediately after the two-hour session, I felt quite spaced out. For example, I had great difficulty deciding what to buy in the supermarket where I went straight afterwards. I did however feel very free physically. Also, I didn't feel pain in my neck but my back still pained me.

An advocate's view of spiritual healing for depression
A 35-year-old female secretary

I have recently come through the break-up of a six-year long relationship. I have had to start all over again as a totally single person finding a new place to live and all that. I felt there was no light at the end of the tunnel for me and I had a lot of self-doubt. Although I was in control of my work life, I felt once I locked the door at night, I became someone else. I had not spoken to anyone in the medical profession about my feelings before I went to the spiritual healer. I felt I really couldn't cope sometimes and I knew that if I went further down that road, I may not be able to get back up again.

Going to the spiritual healer has helped me clear out a lot of channels and given me back faith in myself. She has also knocked down a few barriers for me and said some things that stunned me. Since I started going to her – once every six weeks or so – I am a lot brighter, although I am not completely out of it yet.

She has advised me to have a lavender bath at night as I am a bit of an insomniac. I also have a lavender cushion on my pillow now.

Colour has become more significant for me. I have had my office repainted in a soothing green colour. I used to wear a lot of navy and black. Now, I wear lighter colours. I also have an amethyst which I keep with me to protect me. The comforting thing for me now is knowing that the spiritual healer is there for me when I need her.

The medical view
Evidence for or against spiritual healing is inconclusive.

Choosing a practitioner
The Irish Spiritual Centre, 30 Wicklow St, Dublin 2, has details of some spiritual healers working in Ireland. Tel: 01 6715106. The National Federation of Spiritual Healers in the UK (NFSH) has approximately 8,000 members. Contact details for these spiritual healers working in Ireland and the UK are available from the NFSH at Old Manor Farm Studio, Church St, Sunbury-on-Thames, Middlesex TW16 6RG. Tel: 01932 783164. E-mail: office@nsfh.org.uk

Cost of treatment
The cost of a spiritual healing session is approximately €26/£20.

Useful websites
www.nfsh.org.uk

Western Herbal Medicine

What is it?
Western herbal medicine uses European and Native American plant remedies in the treatment of disease. Most practitioners of Western herbal medicine are medical herbalists and use many of the same diagnostic methods as conventional medical doctors. However, they take a more holistic approach to health, seeking out the underlying cause of the problem for treatment in the belief that the suppression of the symptoms will not rid the body of the disease itself.

Herbal drugs are extracts from the whole plant, as compared to many pharmaceutical drugs that are derived from the active constituent of plants. Herbalists believe that the whole plant contains other substances which work alongside the active constituent (in some cases to modify the side effects) in the treatment of illness.

What are its origins?
Western medical herbalism has its roots in traditional herbalism which was widely practised throughout Europe before allopathic (now conventional) medicine became the standard treatment approach over two hundred years ago. Many modern drugs are derived from the plants used by herbalists and up to 25 per cent of drugs prescribed today are herbal in origin.

Present-day herbal medicine grew out of the practice of herbalism by European immigrants to the United States. There, it was combined with the herbal knowledge of the North American Indians. In the nineteenth century, this hybrid version of herbal medicine came back to the UK and became incorporated into the surviving herbal traditions.

What does it treat?
Western herbal medicine treats many conditions including skin problems, digestive disorders, heart and circulatory problems, gynaecological disorders, allergic responses such as hay fever, arthritis, influenza and stress-related conditions such as insomnia. Herbal medicine is dispensed in the form of tinctures, teas, tablets, capsules and creams. Herbalists generally make up their own prescriptions from fresh and dried herbs.

Several plants and herbs that stimulate the hormones or strong bowel movements or raise blood pressure should be avoided during pregnancy. Medical herbalists advise against self-diagnosis for potentially serious illnesses.

A first-timer's experience
A 47-year-old female nurse
I went to a herbalist because I had very heavy menstrual bleeding. I had previously been to my own doctor who had had a lot of blood tests and scans carried out finding nothing wrong internally. I was left with no other alternative than to have a D & C, so I opted to go to a herbalist instead.

The consultation room was very similar to that of a GP without the queues outside. The herbalist took my blood pressure and asked me a lot of the same questions that a doctor would, except that she spent a lot more time listening to the answers. She also took a detailed medical history, asked me about my diet and if I was using evening primrose oil.

She suggested some adjustments I could make to my diet. Then, she made up a mixture of herbs in front of me and put the liquid in a brown bottle. She asked me to take two teaspoons of this every day for three months. She also gave me five capsules to take one a day for five days and another liquid remedy to take a half an hour before going to bed to help with insomnia. At the end of the consultation, I felt I trusted the herbalist and her professionalism. I thought that even if these remedies didn't do me any good, they wouldn't do me any harm.

An advocate's view of Western herbal medicine and irritable bowel syndrome
A 66-year-old female counsellor
I have had irritable bowel syndrome all my life and have been aware that it is stress-related. Once every few weeks, I would experience pain and bouts of diarrhoea and feel very drained, low in energy and down in spirits afterwards. I didn't think it was something which could be treated and in fact, it took me years to find a name for it. I didn't try the conventional route, but I did discover from experience not to eat acidic foods or highly spiced foods.

Then I saw the name of a medical herbalist (who I initially thought was an orthodox doctor qualified in herbalism) and decided to go to see her. At the consultation, she explained to me all about my condition and the herbs that would bring my bowel back into balance. She advised me to take the liquid herbs three times a day before meals and a little extra prior to an event I anticipated would be stressful.

I found that I had confidence in the medicine and felt it was going to help. I took it consciously with the intent that it would bring my bowel back into balance. There was no sense of a magical instant cure. I had one episode of pain and diarrhoea three weeks after beginning the remedy. Since then, the condition has become much milder and I feel that after having such a pattern throughout my life, I will now be able to keep my bowel in balance by using the herbs indefinitely – in consultation with my herbalist.

The medical view

Herbal medicines have been shown to be helpful when applied topically in otherwise difficult-to-treat cases of eczema and psoriasis. It is important to inform your conventional doctor about any herbal medications you are taking. Likewise, you should inform your alternative practitioner of all conventional medicines you have been prescribed. There is a strong tradition of herbal medicine in Ireland and Britain.

Choosing a practitioner

There are 18 medical herbalists affiliated to the Irish Association of Medical Herbalists. Tel: 091 638183. In the UK, the National Institute of Medical Herbalists has a list of registered practitioners available from 56 Longbrook St, Exeter EX4 6AH. Tel: 01392 426022.

Most medical herbalists practising in Ireland and Britain have completed a four-year training course in the UK and have the letters FNIMH or NIMH after their name which shows that they are either a Fellow or Member of the National Institute of Medical Herbalists.

Cost of treatment

Treatments cost from €26/£20 to €39/£30 for the first visit, plus approximately €20/£15 for two to three weeks supply of herbal medicine. Subsequent visits cost between €15/£12 and €20/£15.

Useful website

www.nimh.org.uk

Yoga

What is it?

Yoga therapy involves individuals learning a set of postures and breathing exercises to relieve specific conditions. These are combined with relaxation and meditation to calm the mind and emotions and heal the spirit. After an initial one-to-one consultation for one hour or more, the client goes away with an individual programme of postures (asanas) and breathing exercises (pranayama) to practise regularly at home.

Follow-up consultations are usually shorter and involve the yoga therapist checking that the client is doing the movements correctly in tandem with the breathing exercises. Attending a regular yoga class (when the teacher is aware of the specific condition being treated) can enhance the effect.

What are its origins?

Yoga is part of the Ayurvedic approach to healthcare from India. The practise of yoga dates back over 3,000 years. It was originally devised as an aid to spiritual enlightenment. Yoga is a Sanskrit word derived from the root *yui,* which means to unite.

What does it treat?

Yoga therapists do not diagnose medical conditions although they will understand such diagnoses. Yoga therapy is complementary to orthodox medicine and is considered a suitable treatment for chronic back pain, arthritis, high blood pressure, rheumatism, depression, insomnia, migraine, asthma and other breathing-related conditions and digestive and menstrual problems. Mothers-to-be are recommended not to start yoga in the first three months of pregnancy.

A first-timer's experience
A 19-year-old female student
I've had back pain for two years as a result of a sports injury. I knew absolutely nothing about yoga before I went to the yoga therapist. In fact, I thought it was for keeping healthy rather than to fix an injury. However, I went along with an open mind. The yoga therapist asked me all about my symptoms, such as when my back hurt most and what aggravated the pain.

Then, she suggested some exercises I could do to strengthen my back. She demonstrated these to me and asked me to do them as well. She also drew diagrams for me to take away. She suggested I begin doing these exercises daily, building up slowly until I was spending about ten minutes a day in all. The session lasted for about an hour.

I hope to do the exercises. I like the idea that it offers me a way of helping myself rather than lying on a bench and have someone else work on me.

An advocate's view of yoga therapy for arthritis
A 66-year-old female full-time carer
When I first went to yoga, I was stressed out to the nines. I was on sedatives for a long time. I couldn't get up in the morning without rolling out of bed, my hips were so stiff and painful.

And, I had lost my sense of humour which – in some ways – was the most difficult aspect of the problem for me.

I had severe arthritis in my neck. I also suffered dizzy attacks due to arthritis in my spine. In fact, I had been suffering for years with osteoarthritis before it was diagnosed. I also suffered from high blood pressure. I really felt if I didn't do something, I would become crippled with pain.

I knew I had to find a better way of life and I needed a break from medication.

I began attending yoga classes and my yoga teacher also made a tape for me which I began to use at home. I find yoga works around your problem and finds its way into it at the same time. Keep breathing, my yoga teacher says and in times of stress now, I always remember to maintain an even breath.

Now, I start every day with a few yoga exercises. I also try to do some throughout the day – say when I'm washing up or standing at the cooker. Yoga helps the circulation, so I don't feel as cold as I used to. As I am a full-time carer, my days are very unpredictable.

I still can't stand for long periods of time and I can't open my hands in the morning without doing simple exercises to help ease them out. At night, I also do yoga exercises before I go to bed. Essentially, yoga has given me back my self-confidence. It has been my life-saver.

The medical view
Yoga is a gentle form of exercise which could help build up the muscles supporting affected joints and help to protect them. In conditions such as arthritis, it would, however, be advisable to avoid maintaining any static yoga position for any period of time, as this could cause pain and stiffness in the joints. The relaxation aspect of the activity may be beneficial in managing the pain component of the condition.

Any activity which causes severe pain is best avoided. Before commencing a course of yoga, it would be wise to seek your doctor's advice.

Choosing a practitioner
Yoga therapists registered with Yoga Therapy Ireland (YTI) can be contacted at 20 Auburn Drive, Killiney, Co. Dublin. Tel: 01 2352120. Yoga therapists in the UK can be contacted through the Yoga Biomedical Trust, 60 Great Ormond St, London WC1N 3HR. Tel: 020 7419 7195. E-mail: yogabio.med@virgin.net.

Yoga therapists usually work with individuals and groups as well as teaching regular yoga classes.

Cost of treatment
Consultations cost €52/£40 per visit.

Useful websites
www.yogatherapyireland.com
www.yogatherapy.org

Glossary

Acute: Short, sharp and quickly over. Acute conditions usually start abruptly, last a few days and either settle or become persistent and long-lasting (see **chronic**).

Allopathic: A term used to refer to conventional or orthodox medicine in which the treatment approach is directed to 'oppose' disease processes.

Ayurveda: A traditional Indian system of medicine which seeks to achieve an optimum balance within the body, mind and spirit. The emphasis is on prevention rather than cure, with strong components of dietary advice and exercise for the body and mind through yoga and meditation.

Chakra: A chakra is an energy centre in the body. There are seven chakras – the crown and brow chakras in the head and five chakras along the spine: the root chakra, the abdominal chakra, the solar plexus chakra, the heart chakra and the throat chakra. Crystal healers work with chakras both in diagnosis and treatment. Yoga practitioners will also connect with these energy centres during postures and meditation.

Chi: Also written as *qi* or *ki* (in Japanese). This is the basic life force or energy as defined by traditional Chinese medicine and its therapeutic offshoots.

Chronic: Long-lasting and persistent. Used in relation to a condition, illness or pain which the patient has for a period of months or years.

D & C: Dilation and curettage, an operation to clear unwanted material from the womb.

Drug interaction: When one drug or medicine changes the effectiveness of another or when the combined dosage increases the toxicity of the medicines taken.

Ergonomic: Having an impact on the working environment of individuals. Ergonomics is the study of the working environment and the measures (for example, well-designed desks, chairs which are positioned correctly for individual needs) which can be taken to optimise this environment in the interests of the users and the task to be completed.

Herbalism: A system of medicine in which extracts from the whole plant are used in the treatment of illness. The theory behind herbalism is that the whole plant contains both the active ingredient required to treat the condition and other constituents which will, for example, improve absorbency and reduce side effects.

Homeopathic: The term used to refer to the system of medicine in which like is treated with like, otherwise known as the Law of Similars.

Immuno-suppressant: Drugs which act on any part of the immune system so as to interfere with the normal reactions to external bacteria or viruses are described as immuno-suppressant drugs.

Manipulation: A series of movements of the joints and spinal vertebrae used by osteopaths and chiropractors in their treatment approach.

Meridian: The pathways or channels along which chi, or energy, travels throughout the body as defined by traditional Chinese medicine. Acupuncture points are situated at specific locations along these pathways.

Musculo-skeletal system: The complex arrangement of muscles and bones in the human body.

Naturopath: A practitioner who sets out to find the underlying causes of disease and use natural cures in treatment. The naturopath is the general term which has more recently given way to specialist categories such as nutritional therapist or massage therapist.

Non-specific: Not related to any particular part or segment of something.

Olfactory: Concerned with smelling.

Oncology: The study of the causes, characteristics and treatment of cancer.

Placebo: An inert substance often used in comparison studies with new drugs; a substance that is medically inactive. The placebo effect refers to an improvement deemed to be due to non-specific aspects of treatment rather than as a result of a direct cause-effect relationship.

Post-operative: The period of time following a surgical intervention.

Remission: A period of time in which the patient shows no or fewer symptoms of a disease or illness which they were previously suffering from.

Shamanic: Practices of healing linked to systems of belief, especially those derived from African tribal customs.

Soft tissue: Internal body parts other than muscle and bone.

Yang: The term used in traditional Chinese medicine diagnosis to describe all characteristics associated with the male natural force. Yang force represents light, heat, dryness and contraction.

Ying: The term used in traditional Chinese medicine diagnosis to describe the opposing yet complementary characteristics to Yang. Ying is associated with female natural force and represents darkness, coldness, moisture and swelling.

Bibliography

Burgess, Jacquie, *Healing with Crystals*, Newleaf, 1997

Clark, Susan, *What Really Works – The insider's guide to natural health, what's best and where to find it*, Thorsons, 2000.

Costigan, Lucy, *Irish Guide to Complementary and Alternative Therapies*, Wolfhound Press, 1997.

Godagama, Dr Shantha, *The Handbook of Ayurveda*, Kylie Cathie, 1997.

Hope-Murray and Tony Pickup, *Healing with Ayurveda*, Gill & Macmillan, 1997.

MacEoin, Beth, *Natural Medicine – A practical guide to family health*, Bloomsbury, 1999.

Olsen, Kristin, *The Encyclopedia of Alternative Healthcare – The complete guide to choices in healing*, Piatkus, 1991.

Quinn, Patricia, *Healing with Nutritional Therapy*, Newleaf, 1998.

Reader's Digest Family Guide to Alternative Medicine, Reader's Digest, 1991.

Sullivan, Karen, *Natural Healthcare for Children*, Piatkus, 2000.

Sustainable Ireland Sourcebook 2000 – Ireland's social, environmental and holistic directory, United Spirits Publications, 2000.

Sutton, Catherine, *Healing with Shiatsu*, Gill & Macmillan, 1997.

Tressider, Andrew, *Lazy Person's Guide to Emotional Healing – Using flower essences successfully*, Newleaf, 2000.

Van Straten, Michael, *The Good Health Directory*, Newleaf, 2000.

Index